Accessing the E-book edition

Using the VitalSource® ebook

Access to the VitalBook™ ebook accompanying this book is via VitalSource® Bookshelf — an ebook reader which allows you to make and share notes and highlights on your ebooks and search across all of the ebooks that you hold on your VitalSource Bookshelf. You can access the ebook online or offline on your smartphone, tablet or PC/Mac and your notes and highlights will automatically stay in sync no matter where you make them.

1. **Create a VitalSource Bookshelf account at** *https://online.vitalsource.com/user/new* or log into your existing account if you already have one.

2. **Redeem the code provided in the panel below to get online access to the ebook.** Log in to Bookshelf and select **Redeem** at the top right of the screen. Enter the redemption code shown on the scratch-off panel below in the **Redeem Code** pop-up and press **Redeem**. Once the code has been redeemed your ebook will download and appear in your library.

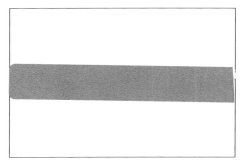

No returns if this code has been revealed.

DOWNLOAD AND READ OFFLINE

To use your ebook offline, download BookShelf to your PC, Mac, iOS device, Android device or Kindle Fire, and log in to your Bookshelf account to access your ebook:

On your PC/Mac

Go to *https://support.vitalsource.com/hc/en-us* and follow the instructions to download the free **VitalSource Bookshelf** app to your PC or Mac and log into your Bookshelf account.

On your iPhone/iPod Touch/iPad

Download the free **VitalSource Bookshelf** App available via the iTunes App Store and log into your Bookshelf account. You can find more information at *https://support.vitalsource.com/hc/en-us/categories/200134217-Bookshelf-for-iOS*

On your Android™ smartphone or tablet

Download the free **VitalSource Bookshelf** App available via Google Play and log into your Bookshelf account. You can find more information at *https://support.vitalsource.com/hc/en-us/categories/200139976-Bookshelf-for-Android-and-Kindle-Fire*

On your Kindle Fire

Download the free **VitalSource Bookshelf** App available from Amazon and log into your Bookshelf account. You can find more information at *https://support.vitalsource.com/hc/en-us/categories/200139976-Bookshelf-for-Android-and-Kindle-Fire*

N.B. The code in the scratch-off panel can only be used once. When you have created a Bookshelf account and redeemed the code you will be able to access the ebook online or offline on your smartphone, tablet or PC/Mac.

SUPPORT

If you have any questions about downloading Bookshelf, creating your account, or accessing and using your ebook edition, please visit *http://support.vitalsource.com/*

OSCEs for the MRCS Part B

OSCEs for the MRCS Part B
A Bailey and Love Revision Guide
Second Edition

Jonathan M. Fishman
BA (Hons), MA (Cantab), BM BCh (Oxon), PhD, MRCS (Eng),
DOHNS (RCS Eng), FRCS (ORL-HNS)
ENT Senior Registrar and Honorary Clinical Lecturer
University College London London,
United Kingdom

Vivian A. Elwell
BA (Hons), MA (Cantab), MBBS, MRCS, FRCS (Neuro. Surg.)
Consultant Neurosurgeon and Spinal Surgeon
Brighton and Sussex University Hospitals NHS Trust
Brighton, United Kingdom

Rajat Chowdhury
BSc (Hons), MA (Oxon), BM BCh (Oxon), MRCS, FRCR, FBIR, PGCME
Consultant Radiologist
Oxford University Hospitals NHS Foundation Trust
Oxford, United Kingdom

All Managing Directors of Insider Medical Ltd

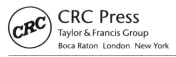

CRC Press
Taylor & Francis Group
Boca Raton London New York

CRC Press is an imprint of the
Taylor & Francis Group, an **informa** business

CRC Press
Taylor & Francis Group
6000 Broken Sound Parkway NW, Suite 300
Boca Raton, FL 33487-2742

© 2018 by Taylor & Francis Group, LLC
CRC Press is an imprint of Taylor & Francis Group, an Informa business

International Standard Book Number-13: 978-1-4987-4156-9 (Paperback)

Visit the Taylor & Francis Web site at
http://www.taylorandfrancis.com

and the CRC Press Web site
http://www.crcpress.com

In loving memory of Dr David S Fishman – we dedicate this book to you.

Contents

Preface

This book has been written as an accompaniment to *Bailey & Love's Short Practice of Surgery* (27th edition) with the Membership of the Royal College of Surgeons examination in mind. It is dedicated to the Membership of the Royal College of Surgeons Part B Objective Structured Clinical Examination, which is the final part of the Intercollegiate Membership of the Royal College of Surgeons examination. This new examination was introduced in the autumn of 2008 and was developed to reflect the changes in postgraduate surgical training in the United Kingdom. This exam is designed and set by the Royal Colleges of Surgeons to test the knowledge, skills and attributes acquired during core surgical training. Successful completion of the Membership of the Royal College of Surgeons will then allow surgical trainees to progress to specialty trainee 3 (ST3) in their chosen subspecialty.

Achieving success in the Membership of the Royal College of Surgeons Objective Structured Clinical Examination requires a thorough basic understanding of clinical medicine, professional examination and technical skills, problem solving and decision making, as well as excellent bedside manner and people skills. It is not difficult to appear hesitant and unintelligent under exam duress, even for the most gifted amongst us. However a precise, structured and systematic approach can easily transform the nervous candidate into one who appears confident, dynamic and multi-dimensional. A planned strategic approach, thus, ensures that candidates are equipped with the essential tools to face any challenge they may face.

The Membership of the Royal College of Surgeons Objective Structured Clinical Examination can be likened to a circuit training course, in that the stations are quick and candidates must immediately switch into their new task at the ring of a bell. It is inevitable that adrenaline is running high but, in our experience, it is those candidates that channel these emotions in a positive way that emerge with a positive Membership of the Royal College of Surgeons Objective Structured Clinical Examination result.

This book is based on our highly successful, 'Insider Medical Membership of the Royal College of Surgeons Part B Objective Structured Clinical Examination Course' (www.insidermedical.co.uk, www.insidermedical.com) and the feedback obtained from over a thousand candidates whom we have taught through these courses. We have, therefore, written this book with the aim of targeting high yield topics that are likely to be faced and offer methods to tackle the challenges that may be posed in the exam. We have drawn from our breadth of experience of teaching at both the undergraduate and postgraduate levels and have identified common pitfalls. We, therefore, also include top tips on getting through those tricky situations, which can often be the fine line between success and failure.

We are confident that this book will assist any trainee surgeon to sail through the Medical Membership of the Royal College of Surgeons Objective Structured Clinical Examination with ease and we hope to make the time taken to prepare for the exam that much more enjoyable and rewarding. Our desired outcome is to secure the future of surgical science and practice, by guiding trainee surgeons in their quest for mastering their art.

Jonathan M Fishman
Vivian A Elwell
Rajat Chowdhury

Acknowledgements

This book would not have been possible without the support of the following individuals: Dr David Fishman, Mrs Wendy Fishman, Dr Galia Fishman, Master James Fishman, Miss Emily Fishman, Mrs Carole Elwell, Dr Nigel Mendoza, Mr and Mrs John Cervieri Jr, Dr and Mrs George Leib, Mr and Mrs Ashit Chowdhury, Dr Madhuchanda Bhattacharyya.

Authors

Jonathan M Fishman, BA (Hons), MA (Cantab), BM BCh (Oxon), PhD, MRCS (Eng), DOHNS (RCS Eng), FRCS (ORL-HNS) is a senior specialty registrar in ENT, a Fellow of the Royal College of Surgeons and Senior Editor for *The Journal of Laryngology & Otology* (Cambridge University Press). He graduated with a 'triple' first class honours degree in Natural Sciences from Sidney Sussex College, University of Cambridge, and completed his clinical training at St John's College, University of Oxford. He has held posts in accident and emergency, ENT, general surgery and neurosurgery, as part of the surgical rotation at St Mary's Hospital, Imperial College, London.
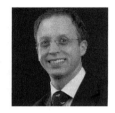

Jonathan has extensive teaching experience and is the primary author of three undergraduate and three postgraduate medical textbooks, including the highly successful *History Taking in Medicine and Surgery* (Pastest Publishing), now in its third edition. He spent part of his medical training at both Harvard University and the NASA Space Center.

Jonathan was awarded the 'Royal Society of Medicine–Wesleyan Trainee of the Year' award in 2012 across all specialties and has been awarded the highly prestigious title of 'Lifelong Honorary Scholar' by the University of Cambridge for his academic excellence. He was awarded a fellowship from the British Association of Plastic Surgeons for research at NASA and from Cambridge University for research at Harvard University. Jonathan has received personal research fellowships from the Academy of Medical Sciences, Medical Research Council, Sparks Children's Charity, the Royal College of Surgeons of England, University College London and the Medical Research Council Centenary Award Scheme. He was awarded a PhD from University College London, in 2013 and is currently honorary clinical lecturer at University College London. He is committed to a career in academic ENT, with a strong emphasis on teaching, research and career development.

Vivian A Elwell, BA Hons., MA (Cantab.), MBBS, MRCS, FRCS (Neuro. Surg.) is a consultant neurosurgeon and spinal surgeon at the Brighton and Sussex University Hospitals NHS Trust. She has a special interest in complex spinal surgery. She obtained her bachelor's degree in biological sciences from Columbia College, Columbia University in New York City, and obtained her master's degree from the University of Cambridge. She then obtained a Bachelor of Medicine and Bachelor of Surgery from the Imperial College School of Medicine, London.
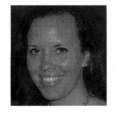

She held posts in accident and emergency, orthopaedics, neurosurgery and general surgery within her surgical rotation at St Mary's Hospital, Imperial College Healthcare NHS Trust, London. She completed her neurosurgical training on the North Thames

Neurosurgery Training Programme, London. Thereafter, she completed the Central London Senior Spinal Fellowship and is committed to coupling her neurosurgical practice with education and research.

Vivian has extensive teaching experience for undergraduate and postgraduate medical education. She is an Instructor for Advanced Trauma Life Support (ATLS®) and Care of the Critically Ill Surgical Patient (CCrISP) Courses. She is an author of five medical textbooks, including *Neurosurgery: The Essential Guide to the Oral and Clinical Neurosurgical Examination* (CRC Press, 2014). She regularly teaches clinical and surgical skills to medical students, doctors and surgical trainees.

Vivian's awards include: the Swinford Edward Silver Medal Prize for her Objective Structured Clinical Examination, the Columbia University Research Fellowship at Columbia College of Physicians and Surgeons the Columbia University King's Crown Gold and Silver Medal Awards, the Kathrine Dulin Folger Cancer Research Fellowship and the 'Who's Who of Young Scientists Prize'. In 2010, she was a finalist for the British Medical Association's Junior Doctor of the Year award. She is noted in 'Who's Who in Science and Engineering' (2011–2012 and 2016–2017).

Rajat Chowdhury, BSc (Hons), MA (Oxon), BM BCh (Oxon), MRCS, FRCR, FBIR, PGCME is a consultant musculoskeletal radiologist at Oxford University Hospitals, a Member of the Royal College of Surgeons and a Fellow of the Royal College of Radiologists. He was awarded an undergraduate Honours degree from University College London, and read medicine at Oxford University. He completed his clinical clinical training at Oxford, Mayo Clinic and Harvard University. He then trained on the surgical rotation at St Mary's Hospital, Imperial College, London, and held posts in accident and emergency, orthopaedics and trauma, cardiothoracic surgery, 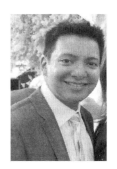 general surgery, and plastic surgery. He then trained in radiology before subspecialising in musculoskeletal radiology, completing his fellowship at Chelsea and Westminster Hospital and an honorary fellowship at the Nuffield Orthopaedic Centre, Oxford.

Rajat has a diverse teaching record. He has taught clinical medicine to students and doctors in Oxford and London, and has tutored biochemistry and genetics to undergraduate students at Oxford University. He was an anatomy demonstrator at the Imperial College School of Medicine, London, and was President of the Queen's College Medical Society, Oxford, and of the Hugh Cairns Surgical Society.

Rajat's academic awards include Oxford University's Bristol Myers Squibb Prize in Cardiology, Radcliffe Infirmary Prize for Surgery, GlaxoSmithKline Medical Fellowship, Warren Scholarship to the University of Toronto and Exhibition Award to Harvard University. He was awarded a NICE Scholarship in 2011 and was National Representative of Leadership and Management at the Academy of Medical Royal Colleges. He is lead author of the undergraduate textbook, *Radiology at a Glance* (Wiley-Blackwell Publishing, 2010) amongst several other titles.

Learn from yesterday, live for today, hope for tomorrow.
The important thing is not to stop questioning.

—Albert Einstein, 1879–1955

Introduction

The MRCS Part B OSCE: The insider's guide to success

Successful completion of the MRCS Part A of the Intercollegiate MRCS examination allows passage to the MRCS Part B OSCE, which is your final stop on the road to becoming a member of one of the Royal Colleges of Surgeons. Furthermore, it marks reaching the landmark to be eligible to enroll on a programme that will train you to be an expert in your chosen sub-specialty. The MRCS OSCE is a truly dynamic exam that demands an equally dynamic response from you to acknowledge your prowess in surgical science and art, as well as your skill and integrity.

The structure of the MRCS Part B OSCE

The MRCS Part B Examination is an Objective Structured Clinical Examination. The MRCS Part B can be likened to a 3½ hour 'circuit course' comprising 18 examined stations each of a 9 minutes' duration. These stations are divided into broad content areas (BCAs):

- Anatomy and surgical pathology (five stations)
- Applied surgical science and critical care (three stations)

These two BCAs are grouped together for the purposes of passing the examination and will be known collectively as 'Applied Knowledge' (eight stations = 160 marks)

- Clinical and procedural skills (six stations)
- Communication skills (four stations)
  - Giving and receiving information
  - History taking

These two BCAs will be grouped together for the purpose of passing the examination and will be known collectively as 'Applied Skills' (10 stations = 200 marks).

In addition, there may be one or more preparation stations and one station that is being pre-tested. Candidates will not be informed which station is being pre-tested.

Each of the 18 examined stations is 'manned'. Some stations will have two examiners and some have only one. In stations with two examiners, each examiner will examine different aspect of your performance.

In addition to the **four broad content areas** mentioned above, **four domains** have been identified to encompass the knowledge, skills, competencies and professional attributes of a competent surgeon. These domains represent the General Medical Council's (GMC) Good Medical Practice (2013) and are assessed in the OSCE, as follows:

- Clinical knowledge and its application
- Clinical and technical skill
- Communication
- Professionalism

MRCS OSCE proposed assessment grid and matrix

Top label: PILOT — Optional – any station as required

Knowledge/Skills broad content area	Sub-area	Station	Examiners required →	Clinical knowledge and its application	Clinical and technical skill	Communication	Professionalism including: Decision making problem solving; situational awareness and judgement; organisation and planning; patient safety	Total mark
SKILLS BROAD CONTENT AREA — Clinical and procedural skills	Procedural skills	Procedural skills - technical	one + assistant		12	8		20
		Procedural skills – patient	one + assistant	4	8	4	4	20
	Physical examination	Physical examination 4	one	4	8	4	4	20
		Physical examination 3	one	4	8	4	4	20
		Physical examination 2	one	4	8	4	4	20
		Physical examination 1	one	4	8	4	4	20
SKILLS BROAD CONTENT AREA — Communication skills	History taking	History taking 2	surgeon + lay	4	4	8	4	20
		History taking 1	surgeon + lay	4	4	8	4	20
	Giving and receiving information	Communicating with colleagues	one	4		8	8	20
		PREPARATION STATION	–					
		Talking with relatives and carers	surgeon + lay	4		12	4	20
		PREPARATION STATION	–					
KNOWLEDGE BROAD CONTENT AREA — Applied surgical science and critical care		Critical care management	one	12	4		4	20
		Interpretation of clinical data	one	12	4		4	20
		Interpretation of data – visual and lab	one	12	4		4	20
KNOWLEDGE BROAD CONTENT AREA — Anatomy and surgical pathology		Surgical pathology and/or microbiology 2	one	20				20
		Surgical pathology 1	one	20				20
		Anatomy 3	one	20				20
		Anatomy 2	one	20				20
		Anatomy 1	one	20				20

Domains tested ↓

These four domains are assessed throughout the 18 stations of the OSCE. Your performance on these domains will not be pass/fail criteria. Domains will be used primarily for structuring the scenarios and mark sheets.

During your 'circuit' each station will be of 9 minutes' duration. In addition, there may be one or more rest or preparation stations and one station that is being pre-tested. The total duration of the OSCE will be approximately 3½ hours; this may vary slightly depending on the time allowed between stations, on the rest break(s) and whether a pre-test station is included.

Each station will have detailed instructions on the outside of the test area about the task to be performed. One minute is allocated for reading the instructions which will also be available within the bay for reference if required. In stations that involve a task followed by interaction with the examiner, there will be an indication of the time allocated for each part. Normally, there will be 6 minutes for the task and 3 minutes for the examiner interaction. A bell will be sounded at this point and the examiner will commence their questioning.

A candidate has 9 minutes to complete each station. If you manage not to complete the task, you will be moved on promptly to the next station (even if you are in the middle of your answer).

Each station is marked out of a total of 20 points. The entire exam is marked out of a total of 360 points.

- Each station is further awarded a global rating for competence marked as
  - Fail
  - Borderline
  - Pass

In order to pass the examination, you must obtain a pass mark in the two aggregated BCAs (knowledge and skills). Using information for the structured mark sheets for each station out of 20, and the global rating for each station, a mark will be calculated out of 160 for knowledge and 200 for skills, that is judged to be the mark required to pass each BCA.

- Knowledge (eight stations) incorporating the BCAs of anatomy and surgical pathology and applied science and critical care.
- Skills (10 stations) incorporating communication skills in giving and receiving information and history taking.

To be awarded a pass in the OSCE, you must pass **EACH** of the two grouped areas at the same sitting.

The mask of a professional

It is clear from the structure of the MRCS Part B OSCE that the experience of completing the exam is like being the only doctor in the hospital and managing the entire surgical division! You are required to manage a trauma call for 1 minute, breaking bad news in clinic the next, suturing a wound seconds later, followed immediately by engaging in academic debate over anatomical prosections, and you have only just started! Furthermore, you are not just trying to maintain your nerve and sanity, you are trying to appear unflustered, confident and in top form every step of the way. This is indeed a very tall order and therefore, one of the most crucial parts of your preparation for this exam is trying to develop a flawless mask of professionalism, composure and control that cannot be removed regardless of the changing challenges that are thrown at you. It is only through maintaining placid composure that you will create the space to have clarity in thought to put together a strategic plan of action and answer questions intelligibly. Many candidates are guilty of the common pitfall of spending disproportionate time on acquiring 'clinical knowledge' and are often careless and lack confidence in their approach. However, equal points are awarded for skill, communication, decision making, organisation and planning. In many ways, the clinical skills (physical examination) stations can be classed in the same genre as the driving test where an exaggerated display of the 'mirror, signal, manoeuvre' protocol is displayed for the benefit of the examiner. In most stations, fastidious attention to basic protocol rituals, such as handwashing and appropriate patient introductions, will not only win favour of the examiners but will also score easy points that could make all the difference between failing and passing comfortably.

Practice makes perfect

The best preparation for this exam is to work with your fellow candidates as a team. You should unashamedly practise and critique each other's performance on systematic physical examinations, practical procedures, viva voce style questioning, as well as discussing and rehearsing communication skills vignettes. You must practise until the step of handwashing, for example, becomes almost an automatic involuntary action. Moving through the exercise of history taking and physical examinations should become swift, smooth and natural so that you can then optimise your efforts on eliciting the salient signs. It is only in this way that you will feel confident to generate an appropriate differential diagnosis for what may seem like a baffling case when under the pressures of extreme exam stress. Examiners will generally not interrupt or prompt you during the examination of patients and so it is up to you to move through the OSCE station picking up all the points available. The best way to achieve this is, therefore, planning every second of your 9-minute routine and practising it to pure perfection. It is only through rigorous rehearsal that a theatrical stage show is perfected for public performance and unforeseen mishaps are managed professionally on opening night. To augment your reading and preparation for this exam, we recommend that you attend our Insider Medical MRCS Part B OSCE Revision Course in London (visit www.insidermedical.co.uk, or www.insidermedical.com for details).

A day in the life of a Specialist Trainee Year 3

An important concept that you should consider is the benchmark your examiners are assessing you against. The MRCS Part B OSCE is a window into the life of you as a potential ST3 to see how you perform and if you are up to the task. You should therefore unofficially rename your preparation for the exam as 'preparing to be an ST3'. You should approach the exam with your 'ST3 hat' on and demonstrate appropriate levels of confidence, gravitas, maturity, safe decision-making and management skills, in addition to your core surgical knowledge and skills. Successful candidates are those who possess flair and finesse, deliver safe logical workups and in essence, portray themselves as a contender to take on the role as a consultant's deputy.

Style over substance

The power of the first impression you create cannot be underestimated and how you look speaks volumes through your non-verbal communication. Modern infection control practices have impacted on dress codes for all healthcare professionals and this now reflects in the exam. Polo shirts and T-shirts are not considered acceptable items of clothing. Best to present yourself as you would for a job interview. Some golden nuggets for portrayal as a responsible, respectable, knowledgeable and safe surgeon include:

Ladies

- Business blouse (arms to be bare below the elbows)
- Minimal jewellery (with the exception of wedding rings) and makeup
- If you have long hair, please tie it back
- Comfortable shoes
- Anti-perspirant and perhaps subtle perfume

Gentlemen

- Business shirt (arms to be bare below the elbows)
- No tie
- Decent, smart haircut
- No jewellery (with the exception of wedding ring)
- Clean and polished shoes
- Anti-perspirant and perhaps subtle aftershave

Mobile phones or other electronic/communication devices must not be carried. They can be left (switched off) with your other property. Carrying such devices can result in disciplinary action.

The dress rehearsal

Revision courses that simulate the exam are excellent to give you a dry run. They can be done at any time but are probably best done when you are nearing the end of your preparation to highlight areas of refinement that can help to further raise your game. You can learn from your own mock exam experience, viewing others in action, and the feedback from the tutors and your colleagues. This is a time to allow others to critique your performance and point out any bad habits that you may be oblivious to. If you attend the course wearing the attire you are likely to be wearing on the day of the actual exam, you will reveal whether your shoes and clothes are comfortable for the 3½ hour OSCE experience.

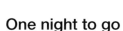

One night to go

Preparation, of course, begins long before the big day. However, on the night before, you should ensure your equipment that you want to take is ready and in order. All equipment that is required for the OSCE will be provided at the exam. However, for familiarity, you might like to take with you the following pieces of equipment:

- Stethoscope
- Tape measure
- Pen
- Pen torch
- Tongue depressor
- Opaque tube (e.g. smartie tube) for transillumination
- Tourniquet (for varicose veins)
- Hat pins (for neurological examination)
- A piece of card for the ulnar nerve examination

Remember, you should test run putting the equipment you want to carry in your assigned pockets and ensure you are still comfortable to conduct the tasks required. Equipment that falls out of your pockets during a physical examination may tarnish your slick image.

You should arrange your travel itinerary as soon as possible and gentlemen should get a smart haircut in the week preceding the exam. On the evening before the big day, you should recheck your itinerary and prepare any paperwork (you will need to take **valid photo ID** (*including your name, signature and photograph*) that must be produced when registering at the exam centre). It is a good idea to prepare your clothes, shoes and bag (including an anti-perspirant if you are prone to anxiety-related perspiration). It is probably not a good idea to experiment with a new restaurant or hit the town but instead set your alarm clock slightly earlier than you comfortably need and then get a good night's rest.

The last few hours

The first test on the big day is not hitting the 'snooze' button when the alarm rings. It is much better to take your time in getting ready than raising your stress levels by oversleeping and then rushing to make the train. Once you're up, it is worth checking the travel updates and then washing and dressing. You should definitely have a proper breakfast because you will need all your energy to be in peak form for the rest of the day. Before you leave, glance in the mirror and tell yourself, you are an ST3!

As a surgical trainee and indeed an ST3, you should conduct yourself professionally and be polite and courteous at all times. After all, you are potentially on display to the examiners before you even arrive at the exam centre, since they may be travelling on the same plane, train or bus as you. Examiners have a habit of sniffing out exam candidates, especially those that have their face buried in this book on the way to the exam!

Top tips for the exam

- Pay particular attention to the briefing before the start of the exam and follow the instructions exactly. You do not want to get noticed by your inability to follow instructions and disorganisation.
- Do not carry your mobile phone/communication device during the exam. This is a disciplinary offence.
- You cannot be too polite and courteous to patients.
- Do not forget to enter your candidate number in unmanned written answer stations.
- You must use the handwash gel before and after every clinical skills station.
- You must listen to the examiner's instructions carefully and follow his or her instructions precisely. If you are at all unclear on what is required of you, do not be afraid to ask the examiner to repeat or rephrase the question.
- Aim to maintain eye contact with the examiners when speaking to them.
- Keep your answers simple and clear – always speak slowly and articulate decisively.
- You will not be interrupted or prompted unless the examiner wants to redirect you. If the examiners are trying to redirect you, do not continue in your current path. You must take the hint and follow their instructions.
- You should execute your well-oiled routine and give an exhibitionary performance. You will not be required to give a running commentary but you may do so if you prefer.
- Summaries must be concise and only contain salient positive and negative findings, followed by a differential diagnosis.
- If you feel one station has not gone particularly well, you must erase it from your mind and stop any rumination in their tracks. It is imperative that you proceed to your next station unflustered and unphased. As an ST3, you may be required to lead a team safely through situations of crisis by maintaining excellent performance – so the show must go on!

The bottom line

Your key for entry into the surgeons' club lies in your ability to think and perform like an ST3!

All the very best of luck!

CHAPTER 1: ANATOMY

INTRODUCTION

Many students find preparing for the anatomy part of the examination a daunting task. It has been many years since you were last in the dissection room and it feels like there is a vast amount of material to learn in a short space of time. It is all too easy to spend all your revision time on anatomy alone, at the expense of other areas of the exam. Although the examiners place a lot of emphasis on anatomy (and rightly so as after all you cannot be a surgeon without knowing your anatomy well), do not neglect other areas of the exam. After all, you must pass all the other areas of the objective structured clinical examination (OSCE) too in order to obtain an overall pass.

As a few top tips:

- Be concise and accurate in your answers.
- Do not say anything you have not been asked about.
- Be systematic and logical.
- Try to apply your answer to surgical practice. The emphasis now is on applied anatomy.

- Do not dig yourself into any holes!
- Remember images that you are asked to comment on in the exam may be normal and the emphasis is on pointing out the key anatomical features, rather than the pathology! So if you are asked to comment on a barium enema do not necessarily go looking for a stricture!

We would recommend that you

- Visit the dissection room prior to the exam and look at some prosections.
- Invest in a good atlas of anatomy.
- Know and be able to demonstrate surface anatomy on a model or patient actor.
- Familiarise yourself with the main bones (osteology).
- Be prepared to be handed 'props' in the exam – bones, prosections, images (e.g. plain radiographs, computed tomography [CT]/magnetic resonance imaging [MRI], contrast studies, angiograms), clinical photographs etc.
- Note that some of the images presented to you in the exam may in fact be normal.
- Know in detail the 'college favourites' which are listed below and also described in this chapter:
  - Skull base, cavernous sinus and pituitary gland
  - Thyroid and parathyroid glands
  - Hand and shoulder joint
  - Blood supply of the stomach
  - Oesophagus and ureters
  - Diaphragm and its openings
  - Portosystemic anastomoses
  - Brachial plexus and axilla
  - Femur, hip and knee joints
  - Heart and coronary artery circulation
  - Surface anatomy (e.g. knee joint, posterior triangle of the neck)

EMBRYOLOGY

Changes at birth

What changes occur at birth?

There are several important changes that take place at birth:

- The urachus (allantois) becomes the single, median umbilical ligament.
- The umbilical arteries become the right and left, medial umbilical ligaments, respectively.
- The left umbilical vein becomes the ligamentum teres (round ligament) in the free edge of the falciform ligament.
- The ductus venosus becomes the ligamentum venosum.

- The ductus arteriosus becomes the ligamentum arteriosum.
- In 2% of cases, the vitello-intestinal duct may persist as a Meckel's diverticulum.
- The foramen ovale in most cases obliterates at birth to become the fossa ovalis, but remains patent into adulthood in some 20% of cases.

Why is this important to know about?

Aberrations of this normal developmental process may lead to pathology:

- Failure of the urachus (that normally connects the bladder to the umbilicus) to obliterate may lead to a urachal fistula, sinus, diverticulum or cyst, often with leakage of urine from the umbilicus.
- Failure of the ductus arteriosus to obliterate at birth leads to a patent ductus arteriosus, resulting in non-cyanotic congenital heart disease.
- In 2% of cases, the vitello-intestinal duct persists as a Meckel's diverticulum with its associated complications.
- In some 20% of cases, the foramen ovale fails to obliterate completely at birth resulting in a patent foramen ovale. This may become the site for paradoxical embolism (where venous thrombus migrates and enters the systemic circulation through a patent foramen ovale), resulting in stroke.

Branchial arches

What are the branchial (pharyngeal) arches, clefts and pouches?

The pharyngeal, or branchial, arches are the mammalian equivalent of the gill arches in fish. In humans, there are five pairs of branchial arches that develop in a cranio-caudal sequence (equivalent to gill arches 1, 2, 3, 4, 6). The fifth branchial arch never forms in humans, or forms as a short-lived rudiment and promptly regresses.

Each arch contains a central cartilaginous element, striated muscle, cranial nerve and aortic arch artery, surrounded by ectoderm on the outside and lined by endoderm.

The arches are separated externally by ectodermally lined branchial clefts and internally by endodermally lined branchial pouches. Branchial cleft derivatives arise from the ectoderm whereas branchial pouches are derived from endoderm.

- The first arch gives rise to the muscles of mastication
- The second arch gives rise to the muscles of facial expression
- The third and fourth arches give rise to the muscles of vocalisation and deglutition
- The sixth arch gives rise to the intrinsic muscles of the larynx

What are the clinical implications?

Certain key features concerning the branchial arches are worth remembering because of their clinical significance:

- The superior parathyroid glands develop from the fourth branchial pouch; the inferior parathyroids, along with the thymus, are third pouch derivatives.

Consequently, the inferior parathyroids may migrate with the thymus down into the mediastinum, hence its liability to end up in unusual positions.

- The tongue is derived from several sources. The anterior two-thirds of the tongue mucosa is a first arch derivative, whereas the posterior one-third is derived from the third and fourth arches. The tongue musculature, in contrast, arises from occipital somite mesoderm. For this reason, the motor and sensory (special taste and somatic touch) nerve fibres of the tongue are carried by separate sets of cranial nerves.
- The thyroid gland arises from between the first and second arch as a diverticulum (thyroglossal duct) which grows downwards leaving the foramen caecum at its origin. Incomplete thyroid descent may give rise to a lingual thyroid, a thyroglossal duct cyst or a pyramidal thyroid lobe. If the thyroid gland descends too far, it may result in a retrosternal goitre.
- Apart from the first branchial cleft (which forms the external ear), the other clefts are normally obliterated by overgrowth of the second pharyngeal arch, enclosing the remaining clefts in a transient, ectoderm-lined, lateral cervical sinus. This space normally disappears rapidly and completely. It may persist in adulthood as a second branchial cleft cyst or fistula.

Name the muscles of mastication, and what are their innervation?

There are four muscles of mastication:

- Temporalis
- Masseter
- Medial pterygoid
- Lateral pterygoid

They are all first branchial arch derivatives and are therefore all innervated by the same nerve (mandibular division of trigeminal, or Vc).

Note: The buccinator muscle is regarded as a muscle of facial expression and is, therefore, a second branchial arch derivative innervated by the facial, or seventh, cranial nerve. This is one of many situations in which a good knowledge of embryology and especially, the branchial arches may help to predict the anatomy.

Gonadal development

Outline the development of the gonads.

During embryonic and fetal life, the testes and the ovaries both descend from their original position at the 10th thoracic level. This explains the long course taken by the gonadal arteries and the site of referred pain from the gonads to the umbilicus (T10 dermatome).

Descent is genetically, hormonally and anatomically regulated and depends on a ligamentous cord known as the gubernaculum. Furthermore, descent of the testis through the inguinal canal into the scrotum depends on an evagination of peritoneum known as the processus vaginalis. This normally obliterates at birth.

How may it go wrong?

Gonadal descent is a complicated process and there are many ways in which it can go wrong. Most commonly, an undescended, or maldescended, testis may occur (cryptorchidism). A patent processus vaginalis may lead to the formation of a congenital hydrocele, or indirect inguinal hernia.

Meckel's diverticulum

What is a Meckel's diverticulum?

A Meckel's diverticulum is the anatomical remnant of the vitello-intestinal duct. In the developing fetus, the vitello-intestinal duct connects the primitive midgut to the yolk sac and also plays a part in intestinal rotation.

The vitello-intestinal duct normally regresses between the 5th and 8th weeks of development, but in 2% of individuals it persists as a remnant of variable length and location, known as a Meckel's diverticulum, named after Johann Friedrich Meckel who first described the embryological basis of this anomaly in the nineteenth century.

Most often it is observed as a 2 inch (5 cm) intestinal diverticulum projecting from the anti-mesenteric wall of the ileum, about 2 feet (60 cm) from the ileo-caecal valve. It is about twice as common in males than in females. However, this useful mnemonic ('the rule of 2s') only holds true in two-thirds of cases; the length of the diverticulum is variable and its site may be more proximal.

What complications might a Meckel's diverticulum undergo?

- It is estimated that 15%–30% individuals with a Meckel's diverticulum develop symptoms from either one of the following:
  - Intestinal obstruction
  - Gastrointestinal bleeding
  - Acute inflammation (Meckel's diverticulitis)
  - Perforation
  - Intussusception
- Its blind end may contain ectopic tissue, namely gastric mucosa (in 10% of cases), liver, pancreatic tissue, carcinoid or lymphoid tissue. This is important because gastric mucosa contains parietal cells that secrete hydrochloric acid. Therefore, ulcers can form within the diverticulum (like a peptic ulcer) causing bleeding.
- Bowel obstruction may be caused by the trapping of part of the small bowel by a fibrous band (that represents a remnant of the vitelline vessels) connecting the diverticulum to the umbilicus. Symptoms may closely mimic appendicitis. Therefore, if a normal-looking appendix is found at laparoscopy, or during an open appendicectomy, it is important to exclude a Meckel's diverticulum as a

cause of the patient's symptoms. Mortality in untreated cases is estimated to be 2.5%–15%.

- Exceptionally, a Meckel's diverticulum may be found in an inguinal or a femoral hernia sac (Littre's hernia).

HEAD, NECK AND VERTEBRAL COLUMN

Thyroid gland

What is the blood supply to the thyroid gland?

The blood supply to the thyroid is by way of the superior thyroid artery (a branch of the external thyroid artery), the inferior thyroid artery (a branch of the thyrocervical trunk of the first part of the subclavian artery) and rarely the small thyroidea ima which arises from the aorta to supply the isthmus. Venous drainage is through the superior and middle thyroid veins to the internal jugular veins and via the inferior thyroid veins to the brachiocephalic veins (usually on the left). This is important to know about when performing thyroid surgery.

Why does the thyroid gland move upwards with swallowing?

The thyroid gland is an endocrine gland that sits as the base of the neck like a bow-tie. It consists of two lateral lobes and an isthmus which is attached via Berry's ligament to the second to fourth tracheal rings (it is not attached to the thyroid cartilage!). The thyroid gland moves upwards with swallowing because

- It is attached to the trachea by Berry's ligament
- It is invested within pre-tracheal fascia

Why is this clinically important?

This is clinically important as it defines a swelling within the neck as being of thyroid origin.

What is the innervation to the muscles of vocalisation?

All the intrinsic muscles of the larynx are supplied by the recurrent laryngeal nerve of the vagus, with the exception of the important cricothyroid muscle, which is supplied by the external branch of the superior laryngeal nerve. Cricothyroid is the muscle which is principally concerned with altering voice pitch by altering the length of the vocal cords. Damage to the superior laryngeal or recurrent laryngeal nerves can occur during thyroid, parathyroid, oesophageal, carotid or aortic arch surgery. Damage to the external branch of the superior laryngeal nerve leads to changes in pitch of the voice whereas damage to the recurrent laryngeal nerve results in a vocal cord palsy leading to hoarseness or even airway compromise (Semon's law).

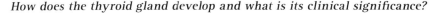

How does the thyroid gland develop and what is its clinical significance?

The embryology of the thyroid gland is clinically extremely important. It descends from the foramen caecum between the anterior two-thirds and posterior third of the tongue via the thyroglossal duct. Before reaching its final position in the neck, it loops under the hyoid bone. An incompletely descended thyroid gland may persist in adult life as a lingual thyroid, pyramidal thyroid lobe or a thyroglossal duct cyst. If it descends too far, it can become a retrosternal thyroid. Thyroglossal duct cysts can become infected and form sinuses or fistulae. In removing a thyroglossal duct, it is important to remove the middle third of the hyoid bone and follow the tract up to the base of the tongue to prevent recurrence (Sistrunk's operation) (Figure 1.1). The ultimobranchial bodies (5th pouch derivatives) give rise to the calcitonin-secreting parafollicular cells ('C cells') of the thyroid gland.

What does the thyroid gland do?

The thyroid gland is stimulated by thyroid-stimulating hormone (TSH) (which is produced from the anterior lobe of the pituitary gland) to produce T3 and T4; hormones which play an important role in basal metabolic rate. The normal thyroid gland produced approximately 90% T4 and 10% T3 but T4 is converted into T3 in the periphery. T3 is the physiologically more active form of thyroxine.

Tongue

What is the innervation of the tongue (sensory and motor)?

Special taste sensation is by way of the chorda tympani division of the facial nerve for the anterior two-thirds of the tongue and the glossopharyngeal nerve for the posterior one-third of the tongue. Taste on the anterior two-thirds of the tongue is therefore commonly lost in a facial nerve (or Bell's) palsy.

Somatic sensation (light touch) is by way of the mandibular division of the trigeminal nerve for the anterior two-thirds of the tongue (lingual nerve) and the glossopharyngeal nerve for the posterior one-third of the tongue.

All the intrinsic and extrinsic (styloglossus, hyoglossus and genioglossus) muscles of the tongue are supplied by the hypoglossal, or 12th cranial nerve, with the exception of the palatoglossus muscle which is supplied by the pharyngeal plexus of nerves (IX, X and sympathetics).

What are the muscles of the tongue?

Intrinsic muscles (wholly within tongue and not attached to bone):

- Longitudinal
- Transverse
- Vertical

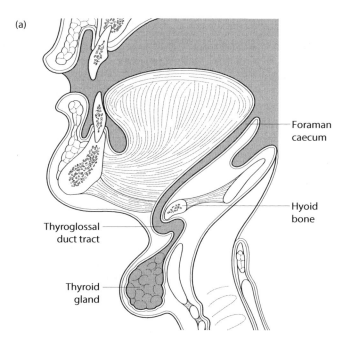

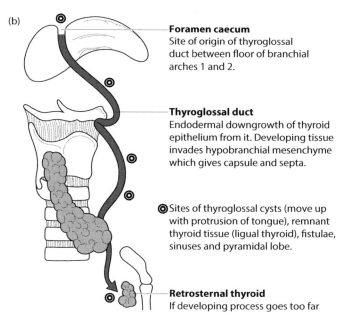

Figure 1.1 (a) Descent of the thyroid gland to its usual position in the neck. (b) Thyroid development.

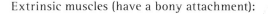

Extrinsic muscles (have a bony attachment):

- Genioglossus
- Styloglossus
- Hyoglossus
- Palatoglossus

What type of epithelium is the tongue lined by?

The tongue is lined by stratified squamous (protective) epithelium as, like the skin, it is subject to 'wear and tear'. Tumours arising from the tongue are therefore typically squamous cell carcinomas.

Parathyroid glands

What are the parathyroid glands?

The parathyroid glands are pinkish/brown glands usually found on the posterior aspect of the thyroid gland. In 90% of individuals, there are four, two on each side, but this varies from two to six. Each weighs about 50 mg and measures 6 × 3 × 2 mm.

How do they develop?

The superior parathyroid glands are fourth branchial pouch (endodermal) derivatives, whereas the inferior parathyroids arise from the third branchial pouch (also endodermal derivatives). The thymus gland is also a third branchial pouch derivative. Therefore, the inferior parathyroid glands may get dragged down with the thymus into the mediastinum making the position of the inferior parathyroid glands highly variable. The superior glands are more constant in position.

What is their blood supply?

All four parathyroid glands are usually supplied by the inferior thyroid artery. A consequence of this is that the inferior thyroid artery should always be preserved during a total thyroidectomy to prevent ischaemia of the parathyroid glands, which would render the patient hypocalcaemic, necessitating lifelong calcium supplementation.

What is their function?

The parathyroid glands secrete parathyroid hormone from chief (or principal) cells. Parathyroid hormone plays an essential role in calcium homeostasis. Calcitonin, on the other hand, is secreted by the parafollicular cells (also known as C-cells or clear cells) of the thyroid gland.

What does a general surgeon need to know about the parathyroids?

The parathyroids can produce too much (hyperparathyroidism) or too little parathyroid hormone (hypoparathyroidism). Hypoparathyroidism usually follows thyroid or parathyroid surgery. Hyerparathyroidism can be primary, secondary or tertiary.

Primary hyperparathyroidism usually results from a parathyroid adenoma (around 90% cases); a benign tumour of usually one (but sometimes more than one) parathyroid gland that leads to the overproduction of parathyroid hormone and hypercalcaemia. Treatment consists of neck exploration and parathyroidectomy. Care must be taken to avoid damaging the recurrent laryngeal nerves. Exposure of the thymus through a midline sternotomy may rarely be necessary given the liability of the inferior parathyroid glands to end up in unusual positions. Less commonly, primary hyperparathyroidism results from multiple adenomas (4% cases of primary hyperparathyroidism), bilateral hyperplasia of the parathyroid glands (5% cases) or rarely a parathyroid carcinoma (1% cases). In the case of bilateral hyperplasia, always think about multiple endocrine neoplasia.

Secondary hyperparathyroidism is usually seen in the setting of chronic renal failure or other causes of vitamin D deficiency (e.g. osteomalacia, malabsorption), where the levels of parathyroid hormone rise in response to a low calcium (remember that the kidney activates vitamin D). Treatment options include subtotal parathyroidectomy (3.5 gland removal), or total parathyroidectomy (four gland removal) with autotransplantation of parathyroid tissue in the latter case.

Tertiary hyperparathyroidism is commonly seen in the setting of renal failure and renal transplant patients and results when the parathyroid glands become autonomously functioning.

	Parathyroid hormone	Serum corrected calcium	Serum phosphate
Primary hyperparathyroidism	↑	↑	↓
Secondary hyperparathyroidism	↑	↓ or normal	↑
Tertiary hyperparathyroidism	↑	↑	↑

What imaging modalities can be helpful in localising parathyroid adenomas pre-operatively?

- Ultrasound scan (USS)
- Sestamibi isotope scanning

Pre-op localisation nowadays enables minimal-access surgery to be carried out.

Skull base

How can the skull base be divided up? (Figure 1.2)

- Anterior cranial fossa
- Middle cranial fossa
- Posterior cranial fossa

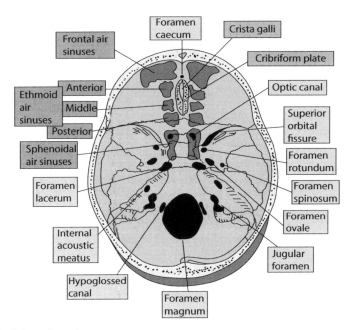

Figure 1.2 Skull base foramina.

What structures run through the optic canal?

- Optic nerve
- Dural sheath
- Ophthalmic artery
- Sympathetics

What runs through the superior orbital fissure?

- Ophthalmic division of trigeminal (Va) – lacrimal, frontal and nasociliary* branches
- Oculomotor nerve (III)*
- Trochlear nerve (IV)
- Abducent nerve (VI)*
- Sympathetic fibres
- Ophthalmic veins
- Branches of middle meningeal and lacrimal arteries

*Through tendinous ring

What runs through the foramen magnum?

- Medulla
- Meninges
- Vertebral arteries with its sympathetic plexus
- Spinal roots of accessory nerve

- Anterior spinal artery (formed from both vertebral arteries)
- Posterior spinal arteries
- Apical ligament of dens
- Tectorial membrane

What runs through the foramen ovale?

- Mandibular division trigeminal (Vc)
- Lesser petrosal nerve
- Accessory meningeal artery

Where is the internal auditory meatus located?

- Petrous temporal bone in the posterior cranial fossa

What structures run through the internal auditory meatus?

- Vestibulo-cochlear (VIII) cranial nerve
- Facial (VII) cranial nerve
- Labyrinthine artery

What is the innervation of the extra-ocular muscles?

The extra-ocular muscles are innervated by the third (oculomotor), fourth (trochlear) and sixth (abducent) cranial nerves. The trochlear nerve and abducent nerve supply only one muscle, that is, the superior oblique muscle and the lateral rectus muscle, respectively. This may be remembered by SO4 and LR6. All the remaining muscles are supplied by the oculomotor nerve – that is, the superior rectus, inferior rectus, inferior oblique and medial rectus are all supplied by the oculomotor, or third, cranial nerve. Injury to any of these cranial nerves (third, fourth or sixth) may result in ophthalmoplegia and diplopia.

The levator palpebrae superioris elevates the eyelid and has a dual innervation from both the oculomotor nerve and sympathetic fibres. The latter innervate a small smooth muscle portion of the levator muscle known as Muller's muscle. The clinical significance of this dual innervation is that a third cranial nerve (oculomotor) palsy, or sympathetic interruption (Horner's syndrome), may result in ptosis.

To distinguish the two, it is essential to lift up the eyelid and inspect the pupil to see if it is enlarged (mydriasis in an oculomotor nerve palsy) or constricted (miosis in a Horner's syndrome). In an oculomotor palsy, the eye points downwards and outwards from the unopposed action of superior oblique and lateral rectus, supplied by the fourth and sixth cranial nerves. Horner's syndrome is associated with hemifacial anhidrosis, flushing symptoms and enophthalmos, in addition to ptosis and miosis.

Posterior triangle of the neck

What are the borders of the posterior triangle of the neck?

- Posterior border of sternocleidomastoid
- Anterior border of trapezius

- Middle one-third of clavicle
- Roof of skin, platysma, investing layer of deep cervical fascia and external jugular vein
- Floor of pre-vertebral fascia covering muscles, subclavian artery, trunks of brachial plexus and cervical plexus

What are the contents of the posterior triangle?

- Nerves – Spinal root accessory and branches of cervical plexus
- Arteries – Superficial (transverse) cervical, suprascapular and occipital
- Veins – Transverse cervical, suprascapular and external jugular
- Muscle – Omohyoid with sling
- Lymph nodes – Level 5

What is the course of the spinal accessory nerve?

The spinal accessory nerve is a branch of the 11th cranial nerve. It has been given the name spinal accessory since it originates from the upper end of the spinal cord (spinal roots, C1–C5). It passes through the foramen magnum and 'hitches a ride' with the cranial accessory nerve originating from the nucleus ambiguus. It passes out of the skull again by way of the jugular foramen. Its function is to supply only two muscles in the neck – the sternocleidomastoid and trapezius muscles.

What is the surface marking of the spinal accessory nerve?

The surface marking of the spinal accessory nerve is important. It traverses the posterior triangle of the neck from one-third of the way down the posterior border of the sternocleidomastoid muscle to one-third of the way up the anterior border of trapezius where it terminates (the 'rule of thirds'). It is vulnerable to iatrogenic injury in procedures that necessitate dissection within the posterior triangle of the neck, such as excision biopsy of a lymph node. In a radical en-bloc lymph node dissection of the neck for malignant disease, the spinal accessory nerve may have to be deliberately sacrificed in order to obtain satisfactory clearance.

What are the consequences of injury to the spinal accessory nerve in the posterior triangle of the neck?

Damage to the spinal accessory nerve in the posterior triangle of the neck leads to a predictive weakness of the trapezius muscle. This results in an inability to shrug the shoulder on the side in which the spinal accessory nerve is affected and may result in winging of the scapula. The sternocleidomastoid muscle is typically spared as the branch to sternocleidomastoid is given off prior to the spinal accessory nerve entering the posterior triangle of the neck. The trapezius muscle also plays a role in hyperabduction of the arm and so activities such as combing one's hair would become more difficult. In the long term, the trapezius palsy (with dropping of the shoulder) may result in a chronic, disabling neuralgia. This may occur as a result of pain from neurological denervation, adhesive capsulitis of the shoulder joint, traction radiculitis of the brachial plexus, or more commonly from fatigue.

Salivary glands

Name the salivary glands.

Major salivary glands:

- Parotid (predominantly serous exocrine secretion)
- Submandibular (mixed mucinous and serous)
- Sublingual (mainly mucinous exocrine secretion)

Minor salivary glands:

- Scattered throughout the oral mucosa and submucosa (labial, buccal, palatoglossal, palatal and lingual)

What important structures lie within the parotid gland?

From superficial to the deep:

- Five terminal branches of the facial nerve (also known as the pes anserinus, or 'goose's foot')
- Retromandibular vein
- External carotid artery
  The mnemonic to remember the contents of the parotid gland is 'facial nerve, retro-mandibular vein, external carotid artery and deep' (FRED). The retromandibular vein is the commonest culprit in a haematoma following parotidectomy.

The facial nerve is the most superficial structure within the parotid gland and hence is extremely vulnerable to injury during parotid surgery. If the retromandibular vein comes into view, the facial nerve has already been severed! A facial nerve monitor should be used throughout and it is important to identify and protect the various branches of the facial nerve, which may be remembered by the mnemonic 'Ten Zulus Baited My Cat' (from top to bottom):

Ten = Temporal branch
Zulus = Zygomatic branch
Baited = Buccal branch
My = Marginal mandibular branch
Cat = Cervical branch

The branches of the facial nerve are also likely to be injured by a malignant tumour of the parotid which is usually highly invasive and quickly involves the facial nerve, causing a facial paralysis.

Where does the parotid duct open?

The duct opens on the mucous membrane of the cheek opposite to the second upper molar tooth.

What is the secreto-motor innervation of the parotid?

The secreto-motor supply to the parotid (for secretion of saliva) is by way of parasympathetic fibres of the glossopharyngeal nerve (lesser petrosal nerve), synapsing in the otic ganglion and relaying onwards to the parotid gland through the auriculotemporal nerve.

What is Frey's syndrome?

A direct consequence of the innervation of the parotid gland is a phenomenon known as Frey's syndrome which may occur, not infrequently, following parotid surgery, or penetrating trauma to the parotid gland. It is caused by misdirected reinnervation of the auriculotemporal nerve fibres to the sweat glands in the facial skin following its injury. The patient may complain of gustatory sweating (i.e. sweating in response to a stimulus intended for saliva production).

What important nerves are at risk during a submandibular gland excision?

- Marginal mandibular division of the facial nerve
- Hypoglossal nerve
- Lingual nerve

How can injury to the marginal mandibular nerve be avoided in a submandibular gland excision?

- Placing the incision two finger breaths beneath the angle of the mandible.
- Raising flaps deep to the investing layer of deep cervical fascia so that the nerve is safe by being pulled laterally in a superficial plane.
- Sectioning the facial vein low in the exposure and reflecting it superiorly thereby drawing the marginal mandibular nerve superiorly away from the gland.
- Gentle traction to prevent stretching of the nerve.
- Intra-capsular dissection of the gland (recommended for benign cases).
- Minimising bleeding around the nerve and avoiding diathermy in close proximity to the nerve.
- Use of the nerve stimulator – Facilitates identification of the marginal mandibular nerve through stimulation or contraction of the depressors to the ipsilateral lower lip.

Cavernous sinus

Define the walls of the cavernous sinus.

The walls of the cavernous sinus may be summarised as follows:

Roof – Anterior and posterior clinoid processes with uncus of temporal lobe and internal carotid artery on it, cranial nerves III and IV into it

Floor – Greater wing of sphenoid

Anterior wall (narrow) – Medial end of superior orbital fissure, ophthalmic veins, orbit

Posterior wall (narrow) – Dura of posterior fossa, superior and inferior petrosal sinuses, peduncle of brain

Medial wall – Dura over sphenoid, sella turcica, pituitary, sphenoidal air sinus

Lateral wall – Dura, temporal lobe, cranial nerves III, IV, Va, Vb in wall (from top to bottom)

Contents – Internal carotid artery (with its associated sympathetic plexus), cranial nerve VI, blood

Note: the optic nerve is *not* contained within the cavernous sinus.

What is meant by the 'danger area' of the face?

The area of facial skin bounded by the upper lip, nose, medial part of cheek and the eye is a potentially dangerous area to have an infection (the so called 'danger area of the face'). An infection in this area may result in thrombosis of the facial vein, with spread of organisms through the inferior ophthalmic vein to the cavernous sinus. This may result in a cavernous sinus thrombosis. By the superficial middle cerebral vein, such thrombosis may spread to the cerebral hemisphere, which may be fatal unless adequately treated with antibiotics.

What hormones does the anterior pituitary gland secrete?

Prolactin, TSH, adrenocorticotropic hormone (ACTH), growth hormone (GH), follicle stimulating hormone (FSH) and luteinizing hormone (LH)

What hormones does the posterior lobe of the pituitary secrete?

Remember using the mnemonic AO (anti-diuretic hormone [ADH]/vasopressin and oxytocin)

Circle of Willis

Draw the circle of Willis and label the different parts (Figure 1.3).

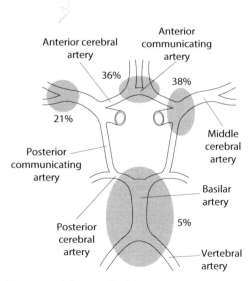

Figure 1.3 Main sites of intra-cranial supraclinoid aneuryms.

Posteriorly:

- At the lower border of the pons, two vertebral arteries combine to form the basilar artery.
- At the upper border of the pons, the basilar artery terminates as right and left posterior cerebral arteries.

Anteriorly:

- Each internal carotid artery gives off an anterior and middle cerebral artery.
- The circle is completed anteriorly by the single, anterior communicating artery which connects the two anterior cerebral arteries.
- The circle is completed posteriorly by the two posterior communicating arteries that connect the posterior cerebral arteries with the internal carotid arteries.

Where are most berry aneurysms situated?

See Chapter 43, 'Cranial neurosurgery', *Bailey & Love's Short Practice of Surgery* 27th edition.

What types of brain haemorrhage are there?

- Subarachnoid haemorrhage – Most commonly due to ruptured berry aneurysms (see above).
- Extradural haematoma – Most commonly due to head injury, resulting in a skull fracture (usually around the pterion of the skull) with rupture of the middle meningeal artery. CT findings include a convex (lens-shaped) haematoma as a result of a collection of blood outside the dura, the latter which is attached to the skull in fixed spaces (see Figure 1.4a).
- Subdural haematoma – Can be acute or chronic, usually resulting from brain atrophy with stretching and rupture of bridging veins across the surface of the brain. Common risk factors include ageing, dementia, bleeding diastheses, anti-coagulants and chronic alcoholism. CT findings include a concave (crescent or lunar-shaped) haematoma which follows the surface of the brain.
- Intra-parenchymal bleed – This is a bleed within the brain substance, usually resulting from hypertension.

Fascial layers of the neck

What does the deep cervical fascia consist of?

- Investing layer of deep cervical fascia
- Pre-tracheal fascia
- Pre-vertebral fascia
- Carotid sheath

What layers does one encounter when a tracheostomy is performed?

- Skin
- Subcutaneous fat
- Superficial fascia with platysma
- Investing layer of deep cervical fascia
- Strap muscles – Sternohyoid muscle is encountered first, followed by sternothyroid

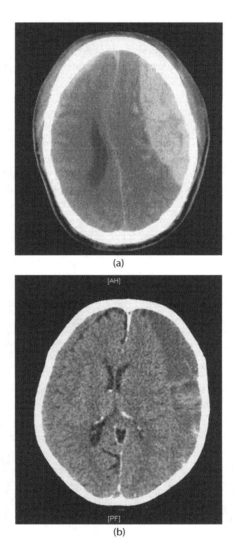

(a)

(b)

Figure 1.4 A large left extradural haematoma – note the convex or lens-shaped haematoma on CT and chronic bilateral subdural haematomas – note the concave or crescent-shaped haematomas on CT.

- Pre-tracheal fascia
- Thyroid isthmus
- Trachea

What does the carotid sheath contain?

- Internal jugular vein
- Carotid artery (common and internal parts)
- Vagus nerve

- Ansa cervicalis embedded within the anterior wall of the sheath overlying the internal jugular vein
- Lymph nodes
- Escaping from the upper part of the carotid sheath are the glossopharyngeal (IX), superior laryngeal branch of vagus (X), spinal accessory (XI) and hypoglossal (XII) nerves

What are the branches of the external carotid artery?

- Superior thyroid
- Superficial temporal
- Maxillary
- Lingual
- Facial
- Ascending pharyngeal
- Posterior auricular
- Occipital

The internal carotid has no branches in the neck and therefore can be easily distinguished from the external carotid artery at surgery (Figure 1.5).

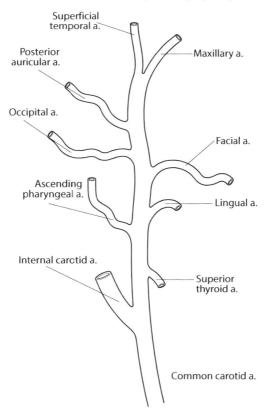

Figure 1.5 Branches of the external carotid artery.

What structures lie at the C6 vertebral level?

- Cricoid cartilage
- Larynx becomes trachea
- Pharynx becomes oesophagus
- Vertebral artery enters foramen transversarium of C6 vertebra
- Inferior thyroid artery and middle thyroid veins cross to thyroid gland
- Middle cervical sympathetic ganglion
- Carotid tubercle of Chassaignac
- Omohyoid (superior belly) crosses carotid sheath

Spinal cord and vertebral column

What type of joint are the inter-vertebral joints?

Secondary cartilaginous joints.

What type of joint is the sacro-iliac joint?

A synovial joint of the plane variety.

What does an inter-vertebral disc consist of?

Between each vertebral body lies an inter-vertebral disc which is made up of an annulus fibrosus of fibrocartilage, with an internal nucleus pulposus consisting of a semi-liquid gelatinous substance derived from the embryonic notochord. With age, the fibrocartilaginous annulus deteriorates and may weaken, often in the lower lumbar region, giving rise to a slipped, or prolapsed, disc. In such cases, the nucleus pulposus is typically extruded posterolaterally.

What is the relationship of the nerve roots to the inter-vertebral discs?

The relationship of the nerve roots to inter-vertebral discs is of great importance. At the level of the L4/5 disc, the fourth lumbar nerve roots within their dural sheath have already emerged from the inter-vertebral foramen and so are not lying low enough to come into contact with the disc. The roots that lie behind the posterolateral part of this disc are those of the fifth lumbar nerve and these are the ones likely to be irritated by the prolapse. Thus, the general rule throughout the vertebral column is that when a disc herniates (usually posterolaterally, rather than in the midline), it may irritate the nerve roots numbered one below the disc. The exception to this rule is in cauda equina syndrome where the disc typically prolapses centrally rather than posterolaterally.

Where does the spinal cord end?

The spinal cord terminates at the level of L1/L2. Below this only nerve roots exist within the vertebral canal (cauda equina). It is therefore safe to perform a lumbar puncture at the level of L3/4 or L4/5. Fortunately for the purpose of a lumbar puncture, the dural sac containing the cerebrospinal fluid (CSF) does not terminate until the level of S2.

What layers does one pass through when performing a lumbar puncture?

- Skin
- Superficial fascia
- Supraspinous ligament
- Inter-spinous ligament
- Ligamentum flavum
- Epidural space (loose areolar tissue containing internal vertebral venous plexus)
- Dura mater
- Arachnoid mater
- CSF in subarachnoid space

THORAX

Breast

Where does the breast lie anatomically?

The base of the breast is fairly constant; from the sternal edge to the midaxillary line and from the second to sixth ribs. Two-thirds of its base overlies pectoralis major and one-third overlaps onto serratus anterior. Contraction of the underlying pectoralis major muscle (by putting one's hands on their hips and pushing in) exacerbates any asymmetry between the breasts (e.g. as a result of a breast cancer) and is a clinically useful manoeuvre.

What is its blood supply?

Blood supply to the breast is mainly derived from the lateral thoracic artery (a branch of the second part of the axillary artery). However, the internal thoracic, thoracoacromial and posterior inter-costal arteries also send branches to the breast.

What is its lymphatic drainage?

The lymphatic drainage of the breast is of considerable anatomical and surgical importance because of the frequent development of breast cancer and the subsequent dissemination of malignant cells along the lymphatics to the neighbouring lymph nodes. Around 75% of the lymphatic drainage of the breast passes to 20–30, or so, axillary lymph nodes. They are usually described as lying in the following groups, which can be remembered by the mnemonic, APICAL:

    A = Anterior (or pectoral) group
    P = Posterior (or subscapular) group
    I = Infraclavicular (or deltopectoral) group
    C = Central group
    A = Apical group
    L = Lateral (or brachial) group

The medial quadrants of the breast (where fortunately cancer is less common) enter the thorax to drain into the internal mammary lymph nodes alongside the internal thoracic artery. Thoracic lymph nodes are difficult, or impossible to treat, but lymph nodes of the axilla can be removed surgically.

The superficial lymphatics of the breast have connections with those of the opposite breast, anterior abdominal wall and supraclavicular lymph nodes. These tend to convey lymph from the breast when the other channels are obstructed by malignant disease, or following their destruction after radiotherapy or surgery.

Lungs

What are the contents of the lung hilum?

- Pulmonary artery
- Main bronchus
- Pulmonary vein
- Bronchial arteries and veins
- Lymph nodes and lymphatic channels
- Autonomics

What is a bronchopulmonary segment?

There are typically 10 anatomically definable bronchopulmonary segments within each lung, each contains a segmental (tertiary) bronchus, segmental artery, segmental vein, lymphatics and autonomic nerves and are separated from their adjacent segments by connective tissue. Each is pyramidal in shape with its apex towards the lung root and its base towards the surface of the lung and is anatomically and functionally separate from the rest. The surgical importance of this is that diseased segments, since they are structural units, can be selectively removed surgically (segmentectomy). Nowadays, this can be performed by video-assisted thoracoscopic surgery (VATS).

How does the right main bronchus differ from the left?

The right bronchus is shorter, wider and more vertical than the left bronchus so that foreign bodies that fall down the trachea are more likely to enter the right bronchus. Furthermore, material aspirated by a supine, comatose or anaesthetised patient would tend to gravitate into the apical segment of the right lower lobe, which is consequently a common site for aspiration pneumonia and abscess formation.

What is the superior limit of the pleura?

The parietal pleura (along with the apex of the lung) projects 2.5 cm above the medial third of the clavicle superiorly. A penetrating wound above the medial end of the clavicle ay therefore involve the apex of the lung resulting in a pneumothorax or collapsed lung. This is most commonly seen as an iatrogenic complication during the insertion of a subclavian (central) venous line. Due to the obliquity of the thoracic inlet, the pleura does not extend above the neck of the first rib, which lies well above the clavicle.

What is the lower limit of the pleura?

It is also important to remember that the lower limit of the pleural reflection, as seen from the back, lies below the medial border of the 12th rib, behind the upper border of the kidney. It is vulnerable to damage here during the removal of the kidney (nephrectomy) through an incision in the loin. Proper identification of the 12th rib is essential to avoid entering the pleural cavity.

Demonstrate the surface anatomy of the pleural linings and lungs.

The reflections (and therefore the surface anatomy) of the pleural linings and lungs may be remembered by the **2, 4, 6, 8, 10, 12 rule**, i.e:

Pleura:

- Starts 2.5 cm above the midpoint of medial one-third clavicle
- Meet in midline at **rib 2**
- Left side diverges at **rib 4** (to make room for the heart)
- Right side continues parasternally to **rib 6**
- Both cross **rib 8** in mid-clavicular line
- Both cross **rib 10** in mid-axillary line
- Both reach posterior chest just below **rib 12**

Lungs:

Below rib 6, the lungs extend to two rib spaces less than pleura (i.e. opposite to rib 6 mid-clavicular line, rib 8 mid-axillary line and rib 10 posteriorly). The parietal pleura extends a further two rib spaces inferiorly than the inferior lung edge to allow space for lung expansion.

Note how the right and left reflections are not identical to one another. On the left, it is displaced by the central position of the heart.

Heart and pericardium

Outline the coronary artery circulation.

There are two principal coronary arteries – the right and left coronary arteries. The right coronary artery originates from the anterior aortic sinus, whereas the left coronary artery originates from the left posterior aortic sinus. The left coronary artery divides into an anterior inter-ventricular (or left anterior descending) artery and circumflex branches. The right coronary artery gives off the posterior inter-ventricular (posterior descending) artery.

The right coronary artery supplies the right atrium and part of the left atrium, sino-atrial node in 60% of cases, right ventricle, posterior part of the inter-ventricular septum and atrio-ventricular node in 80% of cases. The left coronary artery supplies the left atrium, left ventricle, anterior inter-ventricular septum, sino-atrial node in 40% cases and the atrio-ventricular node in 20% of cases.

How many layers does the pericardium consist of?

Three layers:

- Outer fibrous pericardium
- Inner serous pericardium (which comprises both an outer parietal layer and an inner visceral layer)

A small amount of pericardial fluid exists between the visceral and parietal layers of the serous pericardium. This allows the heart to move freely within the pericardial sac.

What are the pericardial sinuses?

Between the parietal and visceral layers, there are two important pericardial sinuses. The transverse sinus lies in between the pulmonary artery and aorta in front and the pulmonary veins and superior vena cava behind. The oblique sinus is a space behind the heart between the left atrium in front and the fibrous pericardium behind, posterior to which lies the oesophagus. The transverse sinus is especially important in cardiac surgery. A digit and ligature can be passed through the transverse sinus and by tightening the ligature; the surgeon can stop the blood flow through the aorta or pulmonary trunk whilst cardiac surgery is performed.

Oesophagus

Describe the course of the oesophagus.

The oesophagus is a segmental muscular tube running from the cricoid ring, at the level of C6, to the cardia of the stomach. It is 25 cm long (with the distance from the upper incisor teeth to the lower oesophageal sphincter being approximately 40 cm). These distances are useful to learn for the purposes of endoscopy. The upper third of the oesophagus consists of skeletal muscle (voluntary muscle which initiates swallowing) but then there is a progressive change to smooth muscle, such that the lower third of the oesophagus consists only of smooth muscle.

What is the blood supply and lymphatic drainage of the oesophagus?

Blood supply and lymphatic drainage is segmental.

- The upper third of the oesophagus is supplied by the inferior thyroid artery and lymphatics drain to the deep cervical group of lymph nodes.
- The middle third of the oesophagus is supplied directly by branches from the descending thoracic aorta and lymphatics drain to the pre-aortic and para-aortic lymph nodes.

- The lower third of the oesophagus is supplied by the left gastric artery and lymphatics drain to the coeliac group of lymph nodes. However, within the oesophageal walls, there are lymphatic channels which enable lymph to pass for long distances within the viscus so that drainage from any given area does not strictly follow the above pattern.

What type of epithelium lines the oesophagus?

The surface epithelium is largely non-keratinizing stratified squamous epithelium. This is normally replaced by columnar epithelium at the gastro-oesophageal junction, but columnar epithelium may line the lower oesophagus. An oesophagus that has the squamocolumnar junction 3 cm or more above the gastro-oesophageal junction is abnormal and called Barrett's oesophagus. This is a metaplastic change taking place in response to acid reflux and is a pre-malignant condition.

Where are the main sites of constrictions along the oesophagus?

- Cricopharyngeus sphincter, 15 cm from the incisor teeth. This is the narrowest part of the oesophagus. The cricopharyngeus sphincter prevents air from entering the oesophagus and stomach and relaxes with the swallowing reflex.
- Where the oesophagus is crossed by the aortic arch, 22 cm from the incisor teeth.
- Where the oesophagus is crossed by the left principal bronchus, 27 cm from the incisor teeth.
- Where the oesophagus passes through the opening in the diaphragm, 38 cm from the incisor teeth.

These measurements are clinically important with regard to the passage of instruments along the oesophagus. They are also sites where swallowed foreign bodies can lodge and where strictures commonly develop.

What factors contribute to the maintenance of the lower oesophageal sphincter?

The lower oesophageal sphincter is not a true anatomical sphincter, but rather a functional one. Maintenance of the lower oesophageal sphincter is largely brought about by the following:

- The effect of the right crus of the diaphragm forming a 'sling' around the lower oesophagus
- The oblique angle the oesophagus takes upon entering the gastric cardia (Angle of His) acting as a 'flap valve' mechanism
- Raised intra-abdominal pressure acting to compress the abdominal part of the oesophagus
- Mucosal rosette (prominent folds at gastro-oesophageal junction)
- Phrenico-oesophageal ligament (fold of connective tissue)
- The effect of gastrin in increasing lower oesophageal sphincter tone
- Antegrade unidirectional peristalsis

- Normal gastric motility and emptying
- Swallowed saliva (lubrication and neutralisation)

A dysfunctional lower oesophageal sphincter may lead to problems, such as gastro-oesophageal reflux disease, hiatus hernia or achalasia.

What is unique about the wall of the oesophagus?

Except for the short intra-abdominal segment of the oesophagus, there is no serosal surface, unlike the rest of the gastrointestinal tract (with the exception of the distal rectum). The consequences of this are two-fold. First, oesophageal anastomoses are particularly prone to leakage, because not only are the anastomoses technically difficult, but also the lack of a peritoneal covering to the oesophagus, with the rather friable oesophageal musculature, means the sutures rely for much of their tensile strength on the mucosa and submucosal layers. Second, because the oesophagus lacks a serosal covering, oesophageal carcinoma encounters few anatomic barriers to local invasion.

What are the characteristic manometric features of achalasia?

- Hypertensive lower oesophageal sphincter
- Non-relaxing lower oesophageal sphincter
- Aperistalsis

Diaphragm

What is the diaphragm?

The diaphragm is a musculotendinous structure composed of outer skeletal muscle fibres and a central tendinous region. It partitions the thoracic from the abdominal cavity and is the main muscle of respiration at rest (accounting for 70% of inspiration at rest).

What is its innervation?

The diaphragm receives motor innervation from the phrenic nerve (C3, C4, C5). (C3, C4, C5 keeps the diaphragm alive!). The diaphragm has no other motor supply other than the phrenic nerve. This is why high cervical spine injuries can be so disastrous and hence the importance of proper cervical spine immobilisation in trauma victims.

The phrenic nerve is two-thirds motor and one-third sensory. The sensory nerve supply to the diaphragmatic parietal pleura and diaphragmatic peritoneum covering the central surfaces of the diaphragm is from the phrenic nerve. The sensory supply to the periphery of the diaphragm is from the lower six inter-costal nerves.

What passes through the various openings in the diaphragm?

A common question!

Vena cava opening (T8)	Inferior vena cava
	Right phrenic nerve
Oesophageal opening (T10)	Oesophagus
	Left and right vagus nerves (RIP = right is posterior)
	Oesophageal branches of left gastric vessels
	Lymphatics from lower one-third oesophagus
Aortic opening (T12)	Aorta
	Azygous and hemiazygos veins
	Thoracic duct
Crura (T12)	Greater, lesser and least splanchnic nerves
Behind medial arcuate ligament	Sympathetic trunks
Behind lateral arcuate ligament	Subcostal (T12) neurovascular bundle

N.B. The **left** phrenic nerve pierces the muscle of the left dome of the diaphragm.

Does the inferior vena cava pass through the muscular or tendinous portion of the diaphragm?

The inferior vena cava passes through the central tendinous portion of the diaphragm at the level of T8. If the vena cava passed through the muscular part of the diaphragm, every time the diaphragm contracts with respiration, it would impede venous return causing syncope.

Thoracic duct

What is the course of the thoracic duct?

- The thoracic duct is 45 cm long and commences at T12 from the cisterna chyli which lies to the right of the aorta.
- It ascends behind the right crus of the diaphragm and to the right of the aorta and oesophagus.
- It crosses the midline to the left, posterior to the oesophagus, at the level of T5.
- In the superior mediastinum, it lies to the left of the oesophagus, posterior to the arch of the aorta and the initial part of the left subclavian artery.
- The thoracic duct lies behind the left common carotid artery, internal jugular vein and vagus nerve.

- It passes over the dome of the left pleura arching anteriorly over the inferior cervical (stellate) ganglion, left vertebral artery, thyrocervical trunk, left subclavian artery and pre-vertebral fascia.
- The pre-vertebral fascia separates the duct from the phrenic nerve and the scalenus anterior muscle.
- The duct lies along the medial edge of scalenus anterior before entering the confluence of the left internal jugular and subclavian veins. It may divide into two or three separate branches, all of which open into the angle between the two veins.
- Valves are present along the duct and encourage the propagation of chyle along the duct.

What areas does it drain?

It drains all lymph below the diaphragm, left thorax and left head and neck regions.

What is the equivalent on the contralateral side?

The equivalent to the thoracic duct on the right is the right lymphatic trunk. This drains on the right into the confluence of the right subclavian and internal jugular veins.

Why do surgeons need to know about the thoracic duct?

Injury to the thoracic duct may occur following trauma, or during insertion of a central venous line. This may result in a chylothorax. The thoracic duct may also be injured in a neck dissection resulting in a chyle leak.

ABDOMEN AND PELVIS

Transpyloric plane of Addison

What important structures traverse the transpyloric plane of Addison?

The transpyloric plane (of Addison) is an important landmark. It lies halfway between the suprasternal notch and the symphysis pubis at the level of L1. It coincides with the following:

- L1 vertebra
- Pylorus of the stomach (hence the name transpyloric)
- Fundus of gallbladder
- Hilum of kidneys
- Hilum of spleen
- Termination of the spinal cord in adults
- Neck of pancreas
- Origin of the portal vein
- Origin of the superior mesenteric artery

- Duodeno-jejunal flexure
- Attachment of transverse mesocolon
- Tip of the ninth costal cartilage

Peritoneal cavity

Where is the epiploic foramen (of Winslow)?

The site at which the greater and lesser sacs of the peritoneal cavity communicate with one other.

What are the boundaries of the epiploic foramen (of Winslow)?

Anteriorly – The lesser omentum with the common bile duct, portal vein and common hepatic artery in its free edge

Posteriorly – Inferior vena cava

Superiorly – The caudate lobe of the liver

Inferiorly – First part of duodenum

Medially – Lesser sac (posterior to stomach)

Laterally – Greater sac

What is its clinical significance?

- It may be the site of internal herniation of bowel.
- Compression of the common hepatic artery in the free edge of the lesser omentum by a carefully placed hand in the epiploic foramen may be a life-saving manoeuvre at laparotomy to control bleeding from the liver (Pringle's manoeuvre).

What three features distinguish large bowel from small bowel?

The following three features distinguish large bowel from small bowel in the cadaver, at laparotomy and on imaging. Large bowel has

- Haustra (also known as sacculations)
- Appendices epiploicae
- Taenia coli

Valvulae conniventes (synonymous with plicae circulares) are a feature of small bowel rather than large bowel.

What spaces are there within the peritoneal cavity?

The most important spaces to recognise are

- Right and left subphrenic (subdiaphragmatic) spaces
- Right subhepatic space (also known as the hepatorenal pouch of Rutherford-Morison).
- Right and left paracolic gutters
- Pelvis

These are potential sites for an intra-abdominal collection. When lying supine, the hepatorenal pouch is the most dependent part of the peritoneal cavity and hence is an area where intra-peritoneal fluid is likely to accumulate in the form of an abscess (or 'collection'). The left subhepatic space is the lesser sac.

How many layers does the greater omentum consist of?

The greater omentum (or gastrocolic omentum) is a double sheet of peritoneum, fused and folded on itself to form an integral structure comprising four layers. The anterior two layers descend from the greater curvature of the stomach where they are continuous with the peritoneum on the anterior and posterior surfaces of the stomach. Posteriorly, they ascend up to the transverse colon where they loosely blend with the peritoneum on the anterior and posterior surfaces of the transverse colon and the transverse mesocolon above it.

What is the blood supply of the greater omentum?

The right and left gastro-epiploic arteries run between the layers of the greater omentum and supply it, close to the greater curvature of the stomach.

How may the lesser sac be approached?

- Through the greater omentum (by incising between the greater curvature of the stomach and the transverse colon and lifting the stomach up)
- Through the lesser omentum
- Through the transverse mesocolon
- Through the epiploic foramen of Winslow
- Through either the gastrosplenic or lienorenal ligaments

Blood supply of the stomach

Draw the blood supply to the stomach (Figure 1.6).

The blood supply to the stomach may be easily remembered by a few simple rules:

Rule 1

The coeliac trunk divides into three main branches, which can be easily remembered by the mnemonic 'left hand side (LHS)':

- Left gastric artery **(L)**
- Common hepatic artery **(H)**
- Splenic artery **(S)**

Rule 2

Divide the stomach up into three main areas:

- Lesser curvature
- Greater curvature
- Fundus

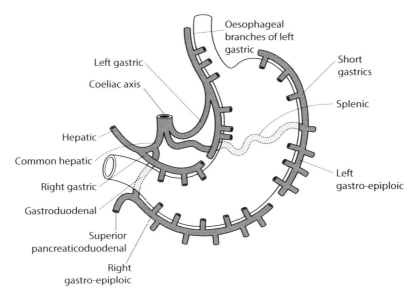

Figure 1.6 Arterial blood supply of the stomach.

Rule 3

The **lesser curvature** is supplied by the **left and right gastric arteries**. The left gastric, as already mentioned, comes directly off the celiac trunk. The right gastric is a branch of the hepatic artery.

Rule 4

The **greater curvature** is supplied by the **right and left gastro-epiploic arteries**. The right gastro-epiploic artery comes off the gastroduodenal artery. The left gastro-epiploic artery comes off the splenic artery.

Rule 5

The **fundus** is supplied by the six, or so, **short gastric arteries** which arise from the splenic artery.

Rule 6

The **gastroduodenal artery** is an important artery. It arises from the **common hepatic artery** and lies posterior to the first part of the duodenum. A posterior placed duodenal ulcer may erode through the duodenal wall into the blood vessel causing catastrophic, life-threatening haemorrhage. Urgent endoscopy or laparotomy may be required to stop the bleeding. A posteriorly placed gastric ulcer may similarly cause life-threatening haemorrhage from the splenic artery.

Gallbladder

What is the surface marking of the gallbladder?

Opposite the tip of the right ninth costal cartilage, that is, where the lateral edge of the right rectus sheath crosses the costal margin. This is an important landmark as it is the site of maximal abdominal tenderness in gallbladder disease.

What is the function of the gallbladder?

The gallbladder has three main functions – it stores bile, concentrates bile (5–20 folds) and adds mucous to the bile secreted by the liver. It has a capacity of about 50 mL. Its mucous membrane is a lax areolar tissue lined with simple columnar epithelium. Under the epithelium, there is a layer of connective tissue, followed by a muscular wall that contracts in response to cholecystokinin, a peptide hormone secreted by the duodenal mucosa in response to the entry of fatty foods into the duodenum.

What is Calot's triangle?

The triangle formed by the liver edge, common hepatic duct and cystic duct. Calot's triangle reliably contains the cystic artery, the cystic lymph node (of Lund), connective tissue and lymphatics. It is important to dissect out this triangle at laparoscopic cholecystectomy in order to successfully identify and ligate the cystic artery prior to the removal of gallbladder.

How does gallstone disease refer pain to the shoulder?

Gallstone disease may refer pain to the right shoulder tip (Kehr's sign). There is an important anatomical explanation underlying this phenomenon. An inflamed or distended gallbladder may irritate the diaphragm which is supplied by the phrenic nerve (C3, 4, 5 keeps the diaphragm alive!). These very same nerve roots also provide sensation to the right shoulder tip by way of the supraclavicular nerves (C3, 4, 5). The body misinterprets the signals that it receives and interprets the pain signals as coming from the right shoulder tip.

What is Courvoisier's Law?

Courvoisier's Law states that in the presence of obstructive jaundice, a palpable gallbladder is unlikely to be due to gallstones. The reason is that gallstones cause chronic inflammation, fibrosis and a shrunken gallbladder. Note, however, that the law does not hold true in reverse (i.e. in the presence of obstructive jaundice an impalpable gallbladder is always due to gallstones) as 50% of dilated gallbladders cannot be palpated on clinical examination, due to patient obesity or because of overlap of the liver.

What factors favour the formation of cholesterol gallstones?

- Bile stasis
- Supersaturation of bile with cholesterol (lithogenic bile)
- Nucleation factors

Portosystemic anastomoses

What are the sites of portosystemic anastomoses?

Portosystemic anastomoses are sites at which the portal venous circulation meets the systemic venous circulation. There are five principal sites where this takes place:

- Lower oesophagus
- Upper anal canal
- Peri-umbilical region of the anterior abdominal wall
- Bare area of the liver
- Retroperitoneum

What is the significance of the portosystemic anastomosis at the lower end of the oesophagus?

The veins from the lower third of the oesophagus drain downwards to the left gastric vein (portal system) and above this level oesophageal veins drain into the azygous and hemiazygous systems (systemic system). Subsequently in portal hypertension dilatations of the veins within the lower end of the oesophagus may take place resulting in oesophageal varices. These can cause life-threatening haemorrhage.

What is the significance of the portosystemic anastomosis within the anterior abdominal wall?

Dilatations of veins within the anterior abdominal wall may result. These are known as caput medusae, because of their resemblance to the hair of the Greek mythological character, Medusa.

What is the significance of the portosystemic anastomosis within the anal canal?

Venous dilatations within the upper end of the anal canal in portal hypertension may lead to the formation of haemorrhoids. However, in practice, they rarely lead to problems and the presence of oesophageal varices are far more significant.

Spleen

What are the anatomical features of the spleen?

The spleen, the largest of the lymphoid organs, lies under the diaphragm on the left side of the abdomen. It may be summarised by 1, 3, 5, 7, 9, 11. That is, it measures 1 × 3 × 5 in., weighs 7 oz. (200 g) and lies beneath the 9th–11th ribs. The spleen lies at the far left extremity of the lesser sac beneath the diaphragm.

It is essential to understand the anatomical relations of the spleen (e.g. the pancreatic tail, stomach, splenic flexure of the colon, left kidney and diaphragm) in order to prevent inadvertent injury to these at splenectomy.

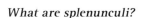

What are splenunculi?

Accessory spleen (splenunculi) represent congenital ectopic splenic tissue and are found in up to 20% of individuals. One or several may be found, usually along the splenic vessels or in the peritoneal attachments. They are rarely larger than 2 cm in diameter.

What are the functions of the spleen?

The functions of the spleen may be summarised by FISH:

- Filtration and removal of old blood cells and encapsulated microorganisms
- Immunological functions (production of IgM and opsonins)
- Storage function (30% of the total platelets are situated within the spleen)
- Haematopoiesis (in the developing fetus)

It has recently been evoked that the spleen has an endocrine function through the production of an immuno-potentiating peptide called tuftsin.

What are the gastrosplenic and lienorenal ligaments?

Two 'pedicles', the gastrosplenic and lienorenal ligaments connect the hilum of the spleen to the greater curvature of the stomach and the anterior surface of the left kidney, respectively. The splenic vessels and pancreatic tail lie in the lienorenal ligament. The short gastric and left gastro-epiploic vessels run in the gastrosplenic ligament.

What organisms are patients susceptible to following splenectomy?

Splenectomized patients with impaired opsonisation are at high risk of post-splenectomy sepsis, especially from encapsulated organisms which evade phagocytosis such as:

- *Haemophilus influenzae*
- *Neisseria meningitidis* (meningococcus)
- *Streptococcus pneumoniae* (pneumococcus)

They may be prevented by administering the relevant vaccinations (Hib, Pneumovax and meningococcal vaccinations, respectively) and giving prophylactic penicillin. Patients are also at risk of malaria (especially *Plasmodium falciparum*).

Adrenal glands

Describe the anatomical features of the adrenal glands?

The adrenal glands lie antero-superior to the upper part of each kidney. They weigh approximately 5 g each and measure 50 mm vertically, 30 mm across and 10 mm thick. They are somewhat asymmetrical, with the right adrenal being pyramidal in shape and left adrenal being crescentic, and lie within their own compartment of (Gerota's) renal fascia. A fascial septum separates the adrenal gland from the kidney which explains why in nephrectomy (removal of the kidney), the latter gland is not usually displaced (or even seen).

What is the blood supply to the adrenal glands?

Each gland, although only weighing a few grams, has three arteries supplying it – a direct branch from the aorta, a branch from the renal artery and a branch from the inferior phrenic artery. This reflects the high metabolic demands of the tissue.

What is the venous drainage of the adrenals?

The single main suprarenal vein drains into the nearest available vessel – on the right, it drains into the inferior vena cava and on the left, directly into the renal vein. The right adrenal gland is tucked medially behind the inferior vena cava. In addition, the right suprarenal vein is particularly short and stubby. Both these features make the inferior vena cava vulnerable to damage in a right adrenalectomy.

What are the different layers of the adrenal gland and what do they produce?

The adrenal gland comprises an outer cortex and an inner medulla, which represent two developmentally and functionally independent endocrine glands within the same anatomical structure. The medulla is derived from the neural crest (ectoderm). It receives preganglionic sympathetic fibres from the greater splanchnic nerve and secretes adrenaline (70%) and noradrenaline (30%). The cortex is derived from mesoderm and consists of three layers or zones. The layers from the surface inwards may be remembered by the mnemonic GFR:

   G = Zona glomerulosa (secretes aldosterone)

   F = Zona fasciculata (secretes cortisol and sex steroids)

   R = Zona reticularis (secretes cortisol and sex steroids)

Appendix

What is the blood supply to the appendix?

The appendicular artery, a branch of the ileo-colic artery which arises from the superior mesenteric artery.

What is the surface landmark of the appendix?

The surface marking of the base of the appendix is situated one-third of the way up the line joining the anterior superior iliac spine to the umbilicus (McBurney's point). This is an important landmark when making an appendicectomy (McBurney's or Gridiron) incision.

Where may the appendix be found?

The position of the free end of the appendix is very variable. The most common, as found at operation, is the retrocaecal or retrocolic position (75% of cases), with the subcaecal or pelvic position next in order of frequency (20% of cases). Less commonly, in 5% of cases, it lies in the pre-ileal or retro-ileal positions, or lies in front of the caecum, or in the right paracolic gutter.

What layers are encountered by the surgeon when performing an appendicectomy?

- Skin
- Subcutaneous tissue (Camper's fascia)
- Scarpa's fascia
- External oblique aponeurosis
- Internal oblique
- Transversus abdominis
- Transversalis fascia
- Pre-peritoneal (extra-peritoneal) fat
- Parietal peritoneum

Why does appendicitis commonly cause peri-umbilical pain?

Afferent nerve fibres concerned with the conduction of visceral pain from the appendix accompany the sympathetic nerves and enter the spinal cord at the level of T10. Consequently, the appendix refers visceral pain to the T10 dermatome which lies at the level of the umbilicus. Only later, when the parietal peritoneum overlying the appendix becomes inflamed, does the pain become more intense and localise to the right iliac fossa in the region of McBurney's point.

Rectum

Where does the rectum begin and end?

The rectum is 12 cm long, starting at the level of S3 and ending at the puborectalis (levator ani-pelvic floor).

Describe the peritoneal reflections of the rectum.

The rectum has no mesentery and is therefore regarded as retroperitoneal. It is covered by peritoneum on its front and sides in its upper third, only on its front in its middle third and the rectum lies below the peritoneal reflection in its lower third. Do not be confused; although the rectum has no mesentery, the visceral pelvic fascia around the rectum is often referred to by surgeons as the mesorectum. The pararectal lymph nodes are found within the mesorectum, which is removed together with the rectum as a package during rectal excision for carcinoma.

What is the blood supply?

Blood supply is by way of the superior rectal (inferior mesenteric), middle rectal (internal iliac) and inferior rectal (internal pudendal) arteries. The venous drainage is as for the arteries. Note, however, that there is a portosystemic anastomosis in the lower rectal and upper anal canal walls, as branches of the superior rectal (portal) and inferior/middle rectal veins (systemic) meet in the external and internal venous plexuses. This may result in haemorrhoids in portal hypertension.

What is the nerve supply to the rectum?

- The rectum receives parasympathetic nerve fibres from the pelvic splanchnic nerves, or nervi erigentes, originating from S2 to S4. It functions to relax the internal sphincter, contract the bowel and transmit a sense of fullness. Note that the vagus nerve only supplies the bowel up to two-thirds along the transverse colon. The whole of the rest of the bowel inferior to this level (the so-called hindgut) receives parasympathetic fibres by way of the pelvic splanchnic nerves.

• Sympathetic supply to the rectum is through the lumbar splanchnics and superior hypogastric plexus. Sympathetics contract the internal sphincter, relax the bowel and transmit visceral pain.

Inguinal canal

What are the boundaries of the inguinal canal?

Anterior wall – Skin, superficial fascia and external oblique (for whole length) Internal oblique for lateral one-third

Posterior wall – Transversalis fascia (for whole length) Conjoint tendon and pectineal (Cooper's) ligament medially

Floor – Inguinal ligament (Poupart's ligament)

Roof – Arching fibres of internal oblique and transversus abdominis which fuse to form the conjoint tendon on the posteromedial aspect of the canal

The deep inguinal ring is a hole in the transversalis fascia and lies a finger breadth above the mid-point of the inguinal ligament (i.e. half way between the anterior superior iliac spine and pubic tubercle).

The superficial inguinal ring is a hole in the external oblique aponeurosis.

What is a hernia?

A hernia is a protrusion of a viscus, or part of a viscus, outwith its normal position.

How can you distinguish a femoral from an inguinal hernia?

An inguinal hernia lies above and medial to the pubic tubercle, whilst a femoral hernia lies below and lateral to the pubic tubercle.

What is the difference between a direct and an indirect inguinal hernia?

A direct hernia passes straight through a weakness in the anterior abdominal wall and passes through the superficial ring only. An indirect hernia passes through both the deep and superficial inguinal rings and thereby passes along the entire length of the inguinal canal. They can be distinguished clinically by placing your hand over the deep ring and asking the patient to cough (deep ring occlusion test). An indirect hernia is controlled at the deep ring, whereas a direct inguinal hernia is not.

At surgery, the neck of an indirect inguinal hernia lies *lateral* to the inferior epigastric artery, whereas the neck of a direct inguinal hernia lies *medial* to the inferior epigastric artery. Occasionally, a pantaloon hernia may occur (with both direct and indirect components).

What is Hasselbach's triangle and what is its surgical importance?

The boundaries of Hasselbach's triangle are

- Medial half of inguinal ligament
- Linea semilunaris (lateral border of rectus abdominis)
- Inferior epigastric artery

Its surgical importance lies in the fact that the triangle is a potentially weak area in the anterior abdominal wall since it is not reinforced by the conjoint tendon. It is responsible for causing direct inguinal hernias.

What are the contents of the spermatic cord?

Apply the 'rule of 3s':

3 constituents – Vas deferens (the round ligament is the female equivalent), lymphatics, obliterated processus vaginalis.
3 nerves – Genital branch of the genitofemoral nerve (motor to cremaster, sensory to cord), ilioinguinal nerve (within the inguinal canal but **outside** the spermatic cord), autonomics.
3 arteries – Testicular artery, artery to the vas (from the superior or inferior vesical artery), cremasteric artery (from the inferior epigastric artery).
3 veins – Pampiniform plexus, vein from vas, cremasteric vein.
3 fascial coverings – External spermatic fascia (derived from external oblique), cremasteric muscle and fascia (derived from internal oblique and transversus abdominis), internal spermatic fascia (derived from transversalis fascia)

Testis

What is the blood supply to the testis?

The testis is supplied by the testicular artery which arises directly from the descending abdominal aorta at the level of approximately L2. The explanation lies in the fact that the testis develops high up on the posterior abdominal wall early in embryonic life. As it descends into the scrotum during development, the testis carries with it the same blood supply that it received whence it was positioned on the posterior abdominal wall (i.e. from the aorta).

What is the venous drainage of the testis?

There is asymmetry between the two sides. On the right side, the testis drains by way of the pampiniform plexus into the inferior vena cava, but the left testis drains into the left renal vein. This may explain why varicoceles are more common on the left side.

What is the lymphatic drainage of the testis?

As a general rule regarding lymphatic drainage, superficial lymphatics (i.e. in sub-cutaneous tissues) tend to run with superficial veins, whereas deep lymphatics run with arteries. The testis, thus, drains lymph to the para-aortic set of lymph nodes, since the testicular artery arises from the aorta. The scrotum, on the other hand, drains to the inguinal group of lymph nodes. The testis, unlike the scrotum, never drains to the inguinal lymph nodes.

The clinical consequence of this is that a testicular carcinoma metastasises to the para-aortic group of lymph nodes and never results in inguinal lymphadenopathy, unless the scrotum is also involved. A scrotal carcinoma, on the other hand, causes inguinal lymphadenopathy.

What is the innervation of the testis?

The testis is supplied by T10 sympathetic nerves. The consequences of this are two-fold. First, it results in testicular pain (trauma, testicular torsion etc.) being referred to the umbilicus (T10 dermatome). Second, the ureters are also supplied by T10 sympathetics. Thus, a renal calculus may refer pain down to the testis, as is seen in classical renal colic.

What layers does the surgeon traverse when operating on a testis?

- Skin
- Subcutaneous tissue (containing dartos muscle)
- Colles' fascia
- External spermatic fascia (external oblique)
- Cremaster muscle and fascia (internal oblique/transverses abdominis)
- Internal spermatic fascia (transversalis)
- Parietal layer of tunica vaginalis
- Visceral layer of tunica vaginalis
- Tunica albuginea of testis

Ureters

What type of muscle do the ureters consist of?

The ureters are segmental muscular tubes, 25 cm long, composed of smooth (involuntary) muscle throughout their entire length.

What type of epithelium lines the ureters?

The ureters are lined by transitional epithelium (urothelium) throughout their length. Transitional epithelium is almost exclusively confined to the urinary tract of mammals where it is highly specialised to accommodate stretch and to withstand the toxicity of the urine.

How may the ureters be identified at surgery so as to prevent inadvertent ligation?

The ureter is characteristically a whitish, non-pulsatile cord, which shows peristaltic activity when gently pinched with forceps (i.e. it vermiculates).

What is the blood supply to the ureters?

Blood supply to the ureters, like the oesophagus, is segmental. The upper third is supplied by the renal arteries, the middle third from branches given off from the descending abdominal aorta and the lower third is supplied by the superior and inferior vesical arteries. Blood supply to the middle third is the most tenuous. Consequently, the middle third of the ureter is most vulnerable to post-operative ischaemia and stricture formation if blood supply to it is endangered by stripping the ureter clean of its surrounding tissue at surgery.

Where do the ureteric constrictions take place?

Along the course of the ureter are three narrowings that often form the site of obstruction in ureteric calculus disease:

- Pelvi-ureteric junction
- Where the ureter crosses the pelvic brim in the region of the bifurcation of the common iliac artery
- Vesico-ureteric junction

The vesico-ureteric junction is the point of narrowest calibre.

What is special about the way in which the ureters enter into the bladder?

In both sexes, the ureters run obliquely through the bladder wall for 1–2 cm before reaching their orifices at the upper lateral angles of the trigone. This forms a flap valve preventing reflux of urine retrogradely back up the ureters. If this flap valve is congenitally deficient, vesico-ureteric reflux results.

UPPER AND LOWER LIMBS

Hip joint

How is stability of the hip joint brought about?

As with all joints, stability is brought about by the way the various bones articulate with one another (through their incongruous surfaces) and through the various ligaments, tendons and muscles that surround the joint.

Stability is achieved largely as a result of the adaptation of the acetabulum and femoral head to one another, with a snug fit of the femoral head into the acetabulum, deepened by the labrum and further reinforced by three ligaments on the outside of the capsule (the iliofemoral, ischiofemoral and pubofemoral ligaments). The iliofemoral ligament (of Bigelow) is the strongest of the three ligaments. The short muscles of the gluteal region are important muscular stabilisers.

Since the hip is such a stable joint, it requires considerable force to become dislocated. When it does occur, it usually dislocates in the setting of a road traffic accident, where typically the hip joint dislocates posteriorly.

What are the important relations of the hip joint?

The hip joint lies deep to the pulsation of the femoral artery at the mid-inguinal point (half way between the anterior superior iliac spine and the symphysis pubis). Pain at this point may indicate pathology originating in the hip joint. Posterior to the hip lies the important sciatic nerve. Consequently, the sciatic nerve is at risk in a posterior surgical approach to the hip, or in a posterior dislocation.

What is the innervation of the hip joint?

The hip joint is innervated by the sciatic, femoral and obturator nerves (Hilton's Law). The knee joint is also innervated by the same nerves. This may explain why hip pathology commonly refers pain to the knee. In a child that presents with a painful knee, always examine the ipsilateral hip joint, in addition to examining the knee, to avoid missing a diseased hip.

What is the blood supply to the femoral head?

The blood supply to the femoral head originates from three important sources:

1. Most importantly, via retinacular vessels that run up from the trochanteric anastomosis and then along the neck of the femur to supply the major part of the head. The trochanteric anastomosis is formed by an anastomosis of the medial and lateral circumflex femoral arteries and the superior and inferior gluteal arteries.

2. From the obturator artery in the ligamentum teres (round ligament). This is usually more important in children.

3. Via the nutrient, or diaphyseal, artery of the femur, originating from the second perforating artery of the profunda femoris artery.

What are the consequences of this?

An intra-capsular fractured neck of the femur may disrupt the retinacular fibres and consequently disrupt the blood flow to the femoral head resulting in avascular necrosis.

What is the Garden classification?

The Garden classification applies to all intra-caspular fractures. Garden 1 and 2 fractures are undisplaced fractures, whilst 3 and 4 are displaced fractures.

> I – Undisplaced, incomplete or impacted fracture
> II – Undisplaced and complete fracture
> III – Complete fracture with partial displacement
> IV – Complete fracture with total displacement

How would you manage an intra-capsular fracture?

Remember the adage 'one, two . . . screw . . . three, four . . . Austin-Moore'. Garden 1 and 2 are generally treated by internal fixation with cannulated screws. Garden 3 and 4 are generally treated with a hemiarthroplasty. The exception is the young patient with a 3 or 4 where the aim is to try and save the hip and therefore open reduction and internal fixation with cannulated screws is preferable in the first instance to avoid multiple hip revisions in the patient's lifetime.

Shoulder joint

What type of joint is the shoulder joint?

The shoulder joint, like the hip joint, is a synovial joint of the ball and socket variety.

List the rotator cuff muscles and what is their innervation?

There are four rotator cuff muscles – these may be remembered by the mnemonic **SITS**:

- Supraspinatus – Suprascapular nerve (C5, 6)
- Infraspinatus – Suprascapular nerve (C5, 6)
- Teres minor – Axillary nerve (C5, 6)
- Subscapularis – Upper and lower subscapular nerves (C5, 6)

What muscles attach to the coracoid process?

- Coracobrachialis
- Pectoralis minor
- Short head of biceps

What important nerve lies in close proximity to the shoulder joint?

It must never be forgotten that the axillary nerve lies in close proximity to the shoulder joint and the surgical neck of the humerus. Consequently, it is vulnerable to injury at the time of a shoulder dislocation, or whilst attempting to reduce the shoulder back into its normal position following a dislocation. It is therefore imperative (from both a clinical and medico-legal point of view) that the integrity of the axillary nerve is documented, both after seeing the patient who has a dislocated shoulder, but also following successful reduction.

Knee joint

What type of joint is the knee joint?

The knee joint is a synovial joint (the largest in the body), of the modified hinge variety.

Describe the cruciate ligaments of the knee joint.

The cruciate ligaments are two very strong ligaments that cross each other within the joint cavity, but are excluded from the synovial cavity by a covering of synovial membrane (they are therefore described as being intra-capsular, but extra-synovial). They are crucial in the sense that they are essential for stability of the knee.

They are named anterior and posterior according to their tibial attachments. Thus, the anterior cruciate ligament is attached to the anterior inter-condylar area of the tibia and runs upwards, backwards and laterally to attach itself to the medial surface of the lateral femoral condyle. The anterior cruciate prevents anterior displacement of the tibia on the femur.

Backward displacement of the tibia on the femur is prevented by the stronger posterior cruciate ligament which runs from the posterior part of the tibial inter-condylar area to the lateral aspect of the medial femoral condyle. The integrity of the latter is therefore important when walking down stairs or downhill. Tears of the anterior cruciate ligament are common in sports injuries; tears, however, of the posterior cruciate ligament are rare since it is much stronger than the anterior cruciate.

Which bursa around the knee communicate with the joint?

Bursae are lubricating devices found wherever skin, muscle or tendon rubs against bone. There are approximately a dozen bursae related to the knee joint. The details are not important, only the salient points. For instance, the supra-patellar bursa communicates with the knee joint. An effusion of the knee may therefore extend some three to four finger breadths above the patella into the supra-patellar pouch. The pre-patellar and infra-patellar bursae do not communicate with the knee joint, but may become inflamed causing a painful bursitis. Inflammation of the pre-patellar bursa is known as housemaid's knee, whereas that of the infra-patellar bursa is called clergyman's knee.

Describe the menisci of the knee joint.

The menisci, or semilunar cartilages, are cresent-shaped laminae of fibrocartilage, the medial being larger and less curved than the lateral. They have an important role in

1. Distributing the load by increasing the congruity of the articulation

2. Contributing to stability of the knee by their physical presence and by acting as providers of proprioceptive feedback

3. Acting as shock absorbers through a 'cushioning' effect

4. Probably assisting in lubrication

The menisci are so effective that if they are removed, the force taken by the articular hyaline cartilage during peak loading increases by about five-fold. Meniscectomy (removal of the menisci), or damage to the menisci, therefore exposes the articular hyaline cartilage to much greater forces than normal and evidence of degenerative osteoarthritis is seen in 75% of patients 10 years after meniscectomy.

The menisci are liable to injury from twisting strains applied to a flexed weight-bearing knee. The medial meniscus is much less mobile than the lateral meniscus (because of its strong attachment to the medial collateral ligament of the knee joint) and therefore cannot as easily accommodate abnormal stresses placed upon it. This, in part, explains why medial meniscal tears are more common than lateral meniscal tears.

What are the boundaries and contents of the popliteal fossa?

Upper lateral – Biceps femoris
Upper medial – Semimembranosus and semitendinosus

Lower lateral – Gastrocnemius (lateral head) and plantaris

Lower medial – Gastrocnemius (medial head)

Floor – Popliteus, capsule, femur

Roof – Short saphenous and communicating veins, lateral sural cutaneous nerve, sural communicating nerve, end of posterior femoral cutaneous nerve and fascia lata

Contents – Popliteal artery and vein (artery is deepest structure within the popliteal fossa and therefore the popliteal pulse is often difficult to palpate), tibial nerve, common fibular nerve, lymph nodes and fat

Femoral triangle

What are the boundaries of the femoral triangle?

The boundaries of the femoral triangle are the inguinal ligament superiorly, the medial border of adductor longus medially and the medial border of sartorius laterally. The roof is fascia lata and the floor is made up of the following muscles: iliacus, psoas, pectineus and adductor longus.

What are the contents of the femoral triangle?

Use the mnemonic **NAVY** (lateral to medial):

N = **Nerve** (femoral) outside the femoral sheath
A = **Artery** (femoral) within the femoral sheath
V = **Vein** (femoral) within the femoral sheath
Y = **Y-fronts** (space most medially – deep inguinal lymph nodes)

What are the boundaries and contents of the femoral canal?

Within the femoral sheath lies the femoral artery, vein and a space most medially known as the femoral canal. The boundaries of the femoral canal are the femoral vein laterally, the lacunar ligament medially, the inguinal ligament anteriorly and the pectineal ligament posteriorly.

Within the space of the femoral canal normally lies extra-peritoneal fat and a lymph node which is often given its eponymous name, Cloquet's lymph node. Cloquet's lymph node drains the lower limb, perineum and anterior abdominal wall inferior to the umbilicus. It may be enlarged (as inguinal lymphadenopathy) in cases of carcinoma and infection at these sites.

The purpose of the femoral canal is to allow the laterally placed femoral vein to expand into it thereby encouraging venous return. However, a piece of bowel or omentum may extend down into the femoral space causing a femoral hernia.

What is the surface anatomical landmark of the femoral artery?

The femoral artery lies at the **mid-inguinal point** (half-way between the anterior superior iliac spine and symphysis pubis), not to be confused with the **mid-point of**

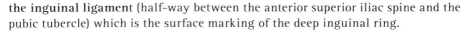
the inguinal ligament (half-way between the anterior superior iliac spine and the pubic tubercle) which is the surface marking of the deep inguinal ring.

This landmark can be used to assess the femoral pulse, but it also provides the clinician with a surface landmark for gaining access to the femoral artery for procedures such as coronary angioplasty and lower limb angiography and embolectomy.

What are the boundaries and contents of the adductor canal?

The adductor canal (also known as the subsartorial canal or Hunter's canal) is an aponeurotic tunnel in the mid-third of the thigh extending from the apex of the femoral triangle proximally through to an opening in the adductor magnus distally (known as the adductor hiatus) to enter the popliteal fossa. Its boundaries are as follows:

> *Roof* – Sartorius and fascia
> *Laterally* – Vastus medialis
> *Medially* – Adductor longus (superiorly) and adductor magnus (inferiorly)
> *Contents* – Superficial femoral artery and femoral vein (latter deep to artery), saphenous nerve, nerve to vastus medialis (in upper part), small branch of posterior division of obturator nerve supplying knee joint, lymphatics

Note that the saphenous nerve and the nerve to vastus medialis do not exit through the adductor hiatus. The femoral artery and vein become the popliteal artery and vein, respectively upon exiting the adductor hiatus. The adductor canal is anatomically narrow and is therefore a common site of turbulent blood flow leading to atherosclerosis.

What is the surface anatomical landmark of the adductor hiatus?

Two-thirds of the way along a line drawn from the anterior superior iliac spine to the adductor tubercle of the femur. Place your stethoscope at this point to auscultate for bruits in distal superficial femoral arterial disease in the claudicant patient since this is the commonest site of lower extremity peripheral vascular disease.

Brachial plexus

What are the root values of the brachial plexus?

The brachial plexus has root values C5–8 and T1. In 10% of cases, the brachial plexus may be either pre-fixed (C4–C8) or post-fixed (C6–T2).

Where are the different parts of the brachial plexus located? (Figure 1.7)

- *Roots* – Exit their respective inter-vertebral foraminae between the scalenus anterior and medius muscles (inter-scalene space)
- *Trunks* – At the base of the posterior triangle of the neck, lying on the first rib posterior to the third part of the subclavian artery
- *Divisions* – Behind the middle third of the clavicle
- *Cords* – In the axilla, in intimate relation to the second part of the axillary artery
- *Terminal Branches* – In relation to the third part of the axillary artery

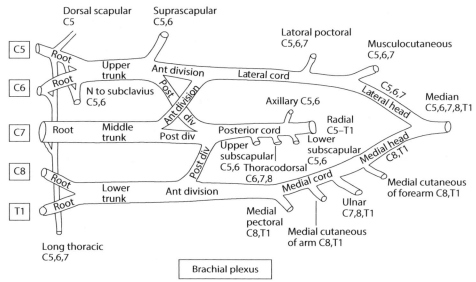

Figure 1.7 The brachial plexus.

The relation of the roots, trunks and divisions of the brachial plexus to the scalene muscles, first rib and clavicle are important. Compression within a fixed space (the thoracic outlet) may lead to symptoms resulting from compression of the brachial plexus and/or nearby vascular structures (subclavian artery and vein). This is known as the thoracic outlet syndrome.

What are the main nerve derivatives of the 'cords' of the brachial plexus?

- *Lateral cord* – Musculocutaneous nerve
- *Medial cord* – Ulnar nerve
- *Posterior cord* – Radial nerve, axillary nerve
- *Medial and lateral cords* – Median nerve

What is the innervation of the serratus anterior muscle?

The serratus anterior muscle is innervated by the long thoracic nerve of Bell (C5, 6, 7). This may be remembered by the old aphorism 'C5, 6, 7 – Bells of heaven'. Denervation of the serratus muscle may result in winging of the scapula.

What are the two main patterns of injury to the brachial plexus?

There are two recognised types of brachial plexus palsy; both usually occur as a result of trauma or obstetric injury. The first follows injury to the upper roots of the brachial plexus (typically C5–C7) and is known as the Erb–Duchenne palsy. The arm typically lies in a waiter's tip position. The second follows injury to the lower roots of the brachial plexus (typically C8, T1) and is known as Klumpke's palsy. The hand in this case typically takes on the position of a 'clawed' hand.

Carpal tunnel

What is the carpal tunnel?

The carpal tunnel is a fibro-osseous tunnel situated on the flexor aspect of the proximal part of the hand and lying between the flexor retinaculum and the carpal bones. Compression of the median nerve within the carpal tunnel is known as carpal tunnel syndrome.

What does the carpal tunnel contain?

It contains the median nerve, together with 10 flexor tendons that include

- Four tendons of flexor digitorum superficialis
- Four tendons of flexor digitorum profundus
- Flexor carpi radialis tendon
- Flexor pollicis longus tendon

N.B. The ulnar artery and nerve do not pass through the carpal tunnel, but instead pass superficial to the carpal tunnel in their own fibro-osseous tunnel, Guyon's canal. The ulnar nerve and artery are therefore unaffected in carpal tunnel syndrome.

Where does the flexor retinaculum attach?

The flexor retinaculum is attached to the tubercle of the scaphoid and pisiform proximally and the hook of the hamate and trapezium distally. Its function is to prevent bow-stringing of the flexor tendons at the wrist.

What muscles does the median nerve innervate in the hand?

The median nerve supplies four muscles in the hand, given by the mnemonic **LOAF**:

    L = Lateral two lumbricals
    O = Opponens pollicis
    A = Abductor pollicis brevis
    F = Flexor pollicis brevis

Would you expect numbness over the thenar eminence in carpal tunnel syndrome?

No, because the palmar cutaneous branch of the median nerve is given off 5 cm proximal to the wrist and then passes superficial to the carpal tunnel.

How would you perform a carpal tunnel decompression?

Can be performed:
- Under general, regional or local anaesthesia
- Open or endoscopic
- With or without a tourniquet

- Check you are doing the right operation, for the right reasons (re-take history, re-examine as necessary and check nerve conduction studies (electrophysiology)

- Fully inform the patient, obtain consent and mark the correct side
- Position the arm extended and fully supinated on an arm board, with the hand held flat by a 'lead hand' retractor
- Standard prep and drape to expose the whole hand
- Incision in line with third web space distal to distal wrist crease
- Extend the incision proximal to the line of first web space (thenar eminence)
- Ensure skin incision is perpendicular to the skin
- Protect the nerve with a Macdonald's elevator
- Check flexor retinaculum is fully released (proximally and distally)
- Irrigation and haemostasis
- Closure 3.0 nylon interrupted vertical mattress sutures
- Mepore dressing and soft, non-constrictive hand bandage
- Encourage elevation of the hand and early mobilisation
- Provide analgesia

What structures are at risk in a carpal tunnel decompression?

- Palmaris longus
- Palmar cutaneous branch of median nerve
- Recurrent motor branch of median nerve
- Superficial branch of the radial artery
- Ulnar artery and nerve
- Palmar arch (superficial and deep)

Anatomical snuffbox

What are the boundaries and contents of the anatomical snuffbox?

Base	From proximal to distal – radial styloid, scaphoid, trapezium, base of first metacarpal
Roof	Skin Fascia
Medially (ulnar side)	Extensor pollicis longus tendon
Laterally (radial side)	Extensor pollicis brevis tendon Abductor pollicis longus tendon
Contents	Cephalic vein (beginning in its roof) Terminal branches of radial nerve (supplying the overlying skin) Radial artery (on its floor)

What is its surgical significance?

- Tenderness within the anatomical snuffbox may indicate a fractured scaphoid bone. This is important to recognise since x-rays are often unaltered in the early stages and if left untreated, there is a high risk of avascular necrosis of the scaphoid (in fact, the proximal scaphoid segment necroses since the scaphoid receives its blood supply from distal to proximal).
- Tendonitis of the abductor pollicis longus and extensor pollicis brevis tendons may occur; this is known as DeQuervain's tenovaginitis stenosans.
- The cephalic vein is almost invariably found in the region of the anatomical snuffbox. This is useful for gaining intra-venous access.

Long saphenous vein

Describe the course of the long saphenous vein.

The long (great) saphenous vein, the longest vein in the body, begins as the upward continuation of the medial marginal vein of the foot. It courses upwards in front of the medial malleolus, in close proximity to the saphenous nerve and runs up to lie a hands-breadth behind the medial border of the patella. It ends by passing through the cribriform fascia that covers the saphenous opening of the fascia lata. Here, it joins the femoral vein at the sapheno-femoral junction, which is located two finger breadths (2–4 cm) below and lateral to the pubic tubercle.

Like all superficial veins of the extremities, the long saphenous vein runs from superficial to deep and contains valves within its lumen. Both these factors prevent the reflux of blood and encourage venous return to the heart.

What is the surgical importance of knowing the anatomy of the long saphenous vein?

1. Varicose veins and their surgical management

2. Venous cut-down as an emergency

3. Harvesting the vein as a graft in vascular and cardiothoracic surgery

What is the course of the short saphenous vein?

The short (small) saphenous vein drains the lateral margin of the foot and lies with the sural nerve behind the lateral malleolus. It passes upwards in the subcutaneous fat to the midline of the calf and pierces the deep fascia to enter the popliteal vein at the sapheno-popliteal junction.

How can you differentiate the long saphenous vein from the femoral vein at the sapheno-femoral junction during varicose vein surgery in order to prevent inadvertently ligating the wrong vessel?

1. The long saphenous vein is more superficial than the femoral vein

2. The long saphenous vein has various tributaries in the region of the saphenous opening including:
   - Superficial circumflex iliac vein
   - Superficial epigastric vein
   - Superficial and deep external pudendal veins

The femoral vein at this level only receives the long saphenous vein itself.

Which nerves may be injured in varicose vein surgery?

- Long saphenous vein surgery – The saphenous nerve (branch of the femoral nerve)
- Short saphenous vein surgery – Sural nerve

CHAPTER 2: SURGICAL PATHOLOGY

Introduction to pathology

Neoplasia

Inflammation

Other topics commonly asked about

INTRODUCTION TO PATHOLOGY

Structuring answers in pathology (as in all bays)

- Define
- Classify
- Amplify

Classifying:

- Congenital versus acquired
- Benign versus malignant
- Malignancies = primary versus secondary (metastatic)
- Aetiology = 'surgical sieve', e.g. INVITED MD (congenital/ genetic + infections, neoplasia, vascular, inflammatory, trauma, endocrine, degenerative, metabolic, drugs & toxins + immune/autoimmune + idiopathic)
- Complications:
  - Immediate/early/late
  - General/systemic versus specific/local
- Effects of tumours = locally invasive versus distant effects (metastatic and non-metastatic/paraneoplastic)

College favourites

- Inflammation – Acute and chronic. Inflammatory bowel disease (IBD).
- Wound healing – Primary, secondary intention, factors affecting wound healing.
- Hypersensitivity reactions.
- Neoplasia – Metaplasia, dysplasia, invasion, metastasis.
- Staging and grading – Tumour, node and metastasis (TNM) classification, Dukes' classification.
- Thrombus, embolus, Virchow's triad.
- Referral to coroner.
- Infections – Tuberculosis (TB)/mycobacteria, human immunodeficiency virus (HIV), clostridia, necrotising fasciitis etc. (see Chapter 3).
- Fistulae, Sinuses, abscess.
- Weird and wonderful – Amyloidosis, pathology specimen pots etc.

NEOPLASIA

Neoplasms

What is a neoplasm?

'An abnormal mass of tissue, the growth of which:

- Is uncoordinated
- Exceeds that of normal tissues
- And which persists in the same excessive manner after cessation of the stimulus which evoked the change (Willis)'

How may neoplasms be classified?

Best to divide into:

- Neoplastic growth disorders
- Non-neoplastic growth disorders (hyperplasia, hypertrophy, hamartoma, metaplasia, dysplasia)

Neoplasms can also be classified as:

- Benign or malignant
- Malignant neoplasms can be further classified as primary or secondary (metastatic)

How may neoplasms be classified according to cell type of origin?

- Classification according to cell type of origin (histogenesis)
- One cell type:
  - Epithelial – Papilloma, adenoma, carcinoma
  - Mensenchymal – Fibroma, lipoma, sarcoma
  - Lymphoma

- More than one cell type from one germ layer
  - Pleomorphic adenoma, fibroadenoma breast, Wilms' tumour
- More than one cell type from more than one germ layer
  - Teratomas (may be benign or malignant)

How may neoplasms be classified according to behaviour?

- Classification according to behaviour – Benign versus Malignant

Benign	Malignant
Non-invasive	Invasive
No metastasis	Capable of metastasis
Resembles tissue of origin (well differentiated)	Variable resemblance to tissue of origin
Slow growing	Rapidly growing
Normal nuclear morphology	Abnormal nuclear morphology
Well circumscribed (pseudocapsule)	Irregular border
Rare necrosis/ulceration	Common necrosis/ulceration

Hyperplasia

What is hyperplasia? Give some examples.

'An increase in size of an organ or tissue through an increase in the number of cells'.

The cells mature to normal size and morphology.

- Physiological examples – Breast, thyroid in pregnancy.
- Pathological examples – Overstimulation – Adrenals in Cushing's, Graves' disease.

Hypertrophy

What is hypertrophy? Give some examples.

'An increase in size of an organ or tissue through an increase in the size of cells'.

There are the same number of cells which mature to normal morphology.

- Physiological examples – Skeletal muscle with exercise, uterus in pregnancy.
- Pathological example – Cardiomyopathy.

Hamartomas

What is a hamartoma? Gives some examples.

'A tumour-like malformation composed of a haphazard arrangement of the different amounts of tissues normally found at that site'.

Grows under normal growth controls of the body.

Examples: Peutz–Jegher's polyps of bowel, haemangiomas.

Metaplasia

What is metaplasia and what is its significance?

- 'A reversible replacement of one fully differentiated cell type with another differentiated cell type'.
- It represents an adaptive change, in response to injury, irritation, altered cell function.
- Reversible.

Significance:

- Greater susceptibility to malignant transformation
- Misdiagnosis will lead to overtreatment

Give three examples of metaplasia.

- Barrett's oesophagus secondary to reflux oesophagitis (change from stratified squamous to glandular, columnar type epithelium)
- Bronchus secondary to cigarette smoking (change from normal respiratory epithelium which is pseudostratified ciliated columnar to stratified squamous)
- Transformation zone of the cervix secondary to human papillomavirus (HPV) (change from normal columnar endocervical epithelium to stratified squamous)
- Carcinoma of the bladder secondary to chronic irritation (calculi/schistosomes)

Dysplasia

What is dysplasia?

'Disordered cellular development characterised by increased mitosis and pleomorphism BUT without the ability to invade through the basement membrane and metastasize to distant sites'.

Severe dysplasia = carcinoma in situ

Carcinomas and sarcomas

What is a carcinoma?

'A malignant tumour of epithelial cells'.

What is a sarcoma?

'A malignant tumour of connective tissue'.

How do they typically spread?

As a general rule, carcinomas typically spread via the lymphatic route; sarcomas typically spread by the haematogenous route. However, there are exceptions to this rule, e.g. follicular thyroid carcinomas spread via the bloodstream to bone.

What makes a tumour malignant?

The key feature of malignancy is

- Invasion through the basement membrane
- Ability to metastasize to distant sites

Metastasis and routes of tumour spread

What is a metastasis?

'The survival and growth of cells that have migrated or have otherwise been transferred from a malignant tumour to a site or sites distant from the primary'.

What are the routes by which tumours spread?

Routes of tumour spread:

- Local invasion
- Lymphatic – Most carcinomas
- Blood – Sarcomas and follicular carcinoma thyroid
- Transcoelomic – Carcinoma stomach, ovary, colon and pancreas, pseudomyxoma peritonei
- Cerebrospinal fluid (CSF) – Central nervous system (CNS) tumours (gliomatosis cerebri)
- Peri-neural – Adenoid cystic parotid
- Iatrogenic – Implantation/seeding during surgery

Which tumours typically spread to bone?

Bone is a favoured site of metastasis from carcinoma of the breast, bronchus, thyroid, kidney, prostate and myeloma.

Cytological and histological features of malignancy

What are the cytological and histological features of malignancy?

Cytological features:

- Hyperchromatism (dark staining nuclei because of increased amounts of DNA)
- Pleomorphism (variance of size and shape of tumour cells and nuclei)
- Cellular atypia
- Increase nuclear-cytoplasmic ratio
- Large and prominent nucleoli
- Increased mitotic index and abnormal mitoses
- Loss of differentiation (anaplastic), failure of cellular maturation

Histological features:

- Loss of normal tissue architecture
- Invasion beyond the basement membrane

- Necrosis (growth outstrips blood supply)
- Haemorrhage (abnormal vascularity)
- Infiltrative borders, with a disordered growth pattern
- Cell shedding (loss of cell–cell cohesion)
- Lymphovascular invasion

Staging and grading

What is staging and grading? What is the difference? Give some examples.

Staging and grading of tumours are the most important prognostic indicators.

- Staging = Extent of growth – based on size and spread of tumour

Examples include:

- TNM system, where T = Tumour size, N = Nodal status, M = Metastasis
- Dukes' (colorectal)
- Breslow thickness, Clark's level (malignant melanoma)

Grading = How well differentiated a tumour is

- Inherent potential for growth
- Based on histological appearance
- Well differentiated (resembles tissue of origin), moderately differentiated, poorly differentiated (anaplastic)

An example is Gleason grading (prostate)

What is Dukes' staging?

Dukes' stage		5 year survival rate (%)
A	In the wall	95–100
B	Through the wall	65–75
C	Lymph node metastases	30–40
D (added later)	Distant metastases	5–10

How is TNM applied to breast cancer?

Primary tumour (T)

Tx   Primary tumour cannot be assessed
T0   No evidence of primary tumour
Tis Carcinoma in situ
T1   Tumour ≤2 cm in greatest dimension
T2   Tumour >2 cm but ≤5 cm in greatest dimension
T3   Tumour >5 cm in greatest dimension
T4   Tumour of any size with direct extension to the chest wall and/or skin

Regional lymph nodes (N)

N0 No regional lymph node metastasis
N1 Metastasis to ipsilateral, mobile axillary lymph nodes
N2 Metastasis to ipsilateral fixed axillary or internal mammary lymph nodes
N3 Metastasis to infra/supraclavicular lymph nodes or to both axillary and internal mammary lymph nodes

Distant metastasis (M)

M0 No clinical or radiological evidence of metastasis
M1 Distant detectable metastasis

Viruses and carcinogenesis

Which viruses cause cancer?

DNA viruses

- Epstein–Barr virus (EBV) – Nasopharyngeal carcinoma (NPC), Burkitt's lymphoma, Hodgkin's lymphoma
- Hep B – Hepatocellular carcinoma (HCC)
- HPV (types 16/18/31) – Cervical cancer, anal carcinoma
- Human herpesvirus 8 (HHV-8) – Kaposi's sarcoma

RNA viruses

- Human T-lymphotropic virus type 1 (HTLV-1) (causes leukaemia/lymphoma in Japan)
- Hep C – HCC

How do viruses cause cancer? (Figure 2.1)

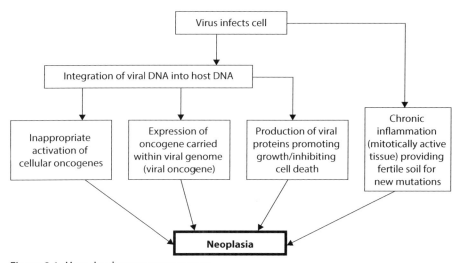

Figure 2.1 How do viruses causes cancer.

Thyroid neoplasms

What types of thyroid neoplasms do you know of?

- Papillary (most common in the United Kingdom)
- Follicular (most common in areas of the world where iodine is deficient)
- Medullary (associated with multiple endocrine neoplasia type 2 [MEN2])
- Anaplastic (worst prognosis)
- Lymphoma

What are the risk factors for thyroid cancer?

- Radiation exposure
- Family history

What is multiple endocrine neoplasia?

A group of related conditions, inherited as autosomal dominant traits, characterised by hyperplasias and/or neoplasms of several endocrine organs. The genetic defect in MEN1 has been linked to a novel gene on chromosome 11 (MENIN gene). MEN2 is clinically and genetically distinct from MEN1 and has been linked to mutations in the RET proto-oncogene located on chromosome 10.

MEN 1 = 3Ps:

- Pituitary adenomas (prolactinomas most commonly)
- Pancreatic islet cell tumours (gastrinomas most commonly)
- Parathyroids (four-gland hyperplasia most commonly)

MEN2a:

- Medullary thyroid carcinoma
- Phaeochromocytoma
- Parathyroid hyperplasia (four-gland hyperplasia most commonly)

MEN2b:

- Medullary thyroid carcinoma
- Phaeochromocytoma
- Marfanoid-type body habitus
- Mucosal neuromatosis

INFLAMMATION

Acute inflammation

What is acute inflammation?

- Acute inflammation = Stereotypical response to tissue injury
- Characterised by calor, dolor, rubor, tumour (heat, pain, redness, swelling)

- +/– functio laesa (loss of function)
- +/– fluor (secretion)

Define the stages.

- Vasodilatation
- Increased vascular permeability
- Diapedesis
- Phagocytosis
- Resolution or progression to chronic inflammation

Name some chemical mediators that participate in acute inflammation.

- Vasoactive amines (histamine, 5-hydroxytryptamine [5-HT]/serotonin)
- Kinin system (bradykinin)
- Complement cascade (C3a, C5a)
- Coagulation cascade and fibrinolytic system
- Arachidonic acid metabolites (leukotrienes, prostaglandins, thromboxane A2)
- Cytokines (interleukins, tumour necrosis factor alpha [TNFα], transforming growth factor beta [TGFβ] etc.)

What are the possible outcomes of acute inflammation?

- Resolution
- Progression to chronic inflammation
- Organisation and repair culminating in scar formation
- Death (meningitis is a good example)
- Abscess formation – This may spontaneously drain to a surface by means of a sinus or fistula

Chronic inflammation

How does chronic inflammation differ from acute inflammation?

Chronic inflammation is defined by the cell types present (macrophages, lymphocytes)

Typically, longer time course than acute inflammation

Causes:

- Persistent infections that evade host defence mechanisms – TB, syphilis, leprosy, *Helicobacter pylori*
- Injurious agent is endogenous – Acid in stomach in peptic ulcer disease
- Persistent/non-degradable toxins – Silica dust, asbestos, lipids in arterial walls (arteriosclerosis)
- The host attacks components of self – Autoimmune diseases – rheumatoid arthritis, Hashimoto's disease
- Host resistance is suppressed – Immunodeficiency states – HIV, malnutrition
- Unknown/Idiopathic – Sarcoidosis, IBD

What are the pathological consequences of chronic inflammation?

- Tissue destruction and scarring
- Malignant transformation
- Amyloidosis (e.g. seen in rheumatoid arthritis, ulcerative colitis)

What is amyloidosis and how is it classified?

Amyloidosis is a condition that results from the aggregation of beta-pleated, insoluble amyloid protein that gets deposited in organs and tissues thereby disrupting their normal function. Amyloidosis may be localised or generalised/systemic and may be primary or secondary to other conditions (e.g. rheumatoid arthritis, IBD). The main subtypes include AL (light chains), AA (inflammatory), Aβ (Alzheimer's disease) and ATTR (familial).

What special histological properties does amyloidosis exhibit?

Amyloid may be stained with Congo red and exhibits 'apple-green birefringence' under plane-polarised light.

Wound healing

What is wound healing?

Wound healing is the process by which tissue restoration of structure and function occurs, with restitution of tissue integrity and tensile strength.

How does a wound heal?

Wound healing can be classified into healing by:

- Primary intention
- Secondary intention (granulation)
- Delayed primary (tertiary) intention

Wounds can heal by resolution (no scar) or by organisation and repair (invariably results in scar tissue).

The stages of wound healing include:

- Haemostasis/coagulation
- Acute inflammation
- Formation of granulation tissue (endothelial cells, fibroblasts, macrophages)
- Angiogenesis
- Epithelialisation, fibroplasia, wound contraction (fibroblasts → myofibroblasts)
- Maturation and remodelling

What factors affect wound healing?

Factors affecting wound healing:

- Local factors – Poor blood supply, haematoma, infection, foreign bodies, surgical technique (excessive wound tension, type of suture material etc.), radiotherapy

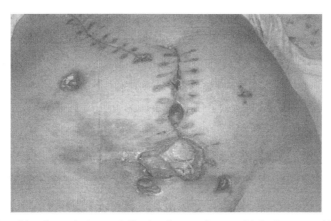

Figure 2.2 Delayed healing relating to infection in a patient on high–dose steroids.

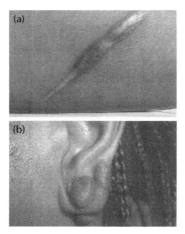

Figure 2.3 (a) Hypertrophic scar after a knife wound. It is raised and stretched, but confined to the boundary of the initial incision. (b) Keloid scar, following an ear–piercing, which is dumbbell shaped, in three dimensions. This became keloid several years after the piercing.

- General/systemic factors – Diabetes mellitus, steroids, immunodeficiency, heart failure, renal failure, liver failure, hypoxia, malnutrition, chemotherapy, malignancy (Figure 2.2)

What is the key difference between hypertrophic and keloid scarring?

In a hypertrophic scar, the scar is confined to the wound margins. They often occur across flexor surfaces and skin creases. In a keloid scar (Greek *kele* = claw + *eidos* = like), the scar extends beyond the wound margins. Keloid scars are more common in patients of Black and Hispanic descent and characteristically occur in the earlobe, chin, neck, shoulder, chest and deltoid regions (Figure 2.3).

Common definitions

What is an abscess?

An abscess is a localised collection of pus surrounded by granulation tissue/fibrous tissue.

What is pus?

A collection of neutrophils, together with dead and dying microorganisms.

What is a sinus?

A blind ending track lined by granulation tissue.

What is a fistula?

An abnormal communication between two epithelial surfaces (or endothelial surfaces e.g. arteriovenous fistula). The commonest fistula is an ear-piercing (Figure 2.4).

What is a stoma?

A surgical opening into a hollow viscus. They can be classified by anatomical site, or output (colostomy, ileostomy, urostomy, tracheostomy, gastrostomy etc.), by indication (temporary vs. permanent) or by the number of openings (end vs. loop).

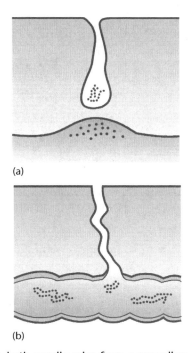

(a)

(b)

Figure 2.4 Sinus and fistula, both usually arise from a preceding abscess. (a) A blind track, in this case a pilonidal abscess. (b) A track connecting two epithelium-lined surfaces, in this case, a colocutaneous fistula from colon to skin.

Fistulae

How may fistulae be classified?

- Congenital (e.g. tracheo-oesophageal fistula) versus acquired
- Aetiology (infections, inflammation, malignancy, radiotherapy etc.)
- Internal versus external
- Simple versus complex
- Anatomical – By site – (e.g. entero-enteric, entero-cutaneous, colo-vaginal, vesico-colic)
- Physiological – High output (>500 mL/day) versus low output

What factors prevent an intestinal fistula from healing spontaneously?

- Distal obstruction
- Malignancy
- Foreign body
- Associated undrained infection
- Radiation injury to tissues
- Underlying inflammatory condition (e.g. Crohn's disease)
- Mucocutaneous continuity
- High output
- Malnutrition

How are fistulae managed?

SNAP!

- <u>S</u>epsis control
- <u>N</u>utritional support
- <u>A</u>natomical assessment, <u>A</u>dequate fluid and electrolyte replacement
- <u>P</u>lan, <u>P</u>rotect skin to prevent excoriation

  Sixty per cent should close spontaneously within 1 month with conservative measures when the sepsis is controlled and distal obstruction has been relieved (Figure 2.5).

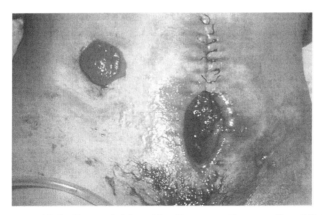

Figure 2.5 Major wound infection and delayed healing presenting as a faecal fistula in a patient with Crohn's disease.

Inflammatory bowel disease

What are the macroscopic and microscopic differences between Crohn's disease and ulcerative colitis?

Inflammatory bowel disease

Inflammatory bowel disease can be classified into:

- Crohn's disease
- Ulcerative colitis
- Indeterminate colitis

What are the extra-intestinal manifestations of IBD?

- Integument – Clubbing, erythema nodosum, pyoderma gangrenosum, aphthous ulcers
- Eyes – Conjunctivitis, episcleritis, scleritis, anterior uveitis
- Liver and biliary tree – Fatty liver, chronic active hepatitis, cirrhosis, gallstones, primary sclerosing cholangitis, cholangiocarcinoma
- Renal tract – Calculi
- Joints – Peripheral arthopathy, sacroiliitis, ankylosing spondylitis
- Amyloidosis

Crohn's	Ulcerative colitis
Anywhere in the gastrointestinal tract	Rectum
'Skip' lesions	Confined to colon
Rectal sparing	Contiguous disease
Full thickness/transmural	+/– Backwash ileitis
Fat wrapping	Mucosal disease
Deep fissures	Pseudopolyps
Fistulae, sinuses	No granulomas
Strictures → Obstruction	Crypt abscesses (UC>CD)
Non-caseating granulomas (~60%)	'Lead pipe' colon
'Cobblestone' mucosa Crypt abscesses (UC>CD)	Dysplasia

Granulomas

What is a granuloma? Give some examples.

A granuloma is a focal area of chronic inflammation. It consists of a microscopic aggregation of activated macrophages that are transformed into epithelium-like cells, surrounded by a collar of mononuclear leukocytes, principally lymphocytes and plasma cells.

Granulomas can be classified into caseating (e.g. TB) versus non-caseating granulomas (sarcoid, Wegener's granulomatosis, Crohn's disease, primary biliary cirrhosis [PBC])

Causes:

- Infections – TB, leprosy, syphilis, actinomycosis
- Inflammation – Sarcoidosis, Crohn's disease, PBC, Wegener's granulomatosis
- Foreign bodies – Beryllium, silicosis, talc, sutures
- Malignancy (e.g. Hodgkin's lymphoma)

OTHER TOPICS COMMONLY ASKED ABOUT

Aneurysms

What is an aneurysm? How are they classified?

An abnormal, permanent, localised dilatation of a blood vessel, to 1.5–2× its normal diameter.

They may be classified by:

- Aetiology (atherosclerotic, inflammatory etc.)
- Congenital versus acquired
- True versus false (pseudoaneurysm)
- Site (e.g. thoracic, abdominal, intracranial)
- Size (giant aneurysms, berry)
- Shape (fusiform, saccular, dissecting etc.)

What are the complications of aneurysms?

- Rupture
- Thrombosis
- Embolism
- Local compressive effects
- Infection (mycotic)
- Fistula (e.g. aorto-enteric fistula) (Figure 2.6)

Polyps

What is a polyp? Name some different types.

A polyp = A pedunculated mass of tissue arising from an epithelial surface.

They can be classified into:

- Non-neoplastic polyps (hyperplastic [also known as metaplastic], hamartomatous, inflammatory pseudopolyps, lymphoid hyperplasia)

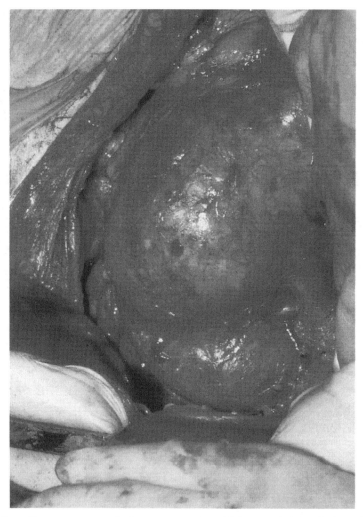

Figure 2.6 Operative appearance of a large, non-ruptured infra-renal abdominal aortic aneurysm.

- Neoplastic polyps (tubular, tubulo-villous, villous). In terms of frequency: tubular (65%–80% of cases) > tubulo-villous (10%–25%) > villous (5%–10%). In terms of malignant potential: villous (40% risk of harbouring cancer) > tubulo-villous (22% risk of cancer) > tubular (5% risk of cancer).

What complications might polyps undergo?

- Malignant transformation
- Ulceration

- Bleeding
- Infection
- Intussusception
- Protein and potassium loss

Diverticula

What is a diverticulum? How are they classified?

A diverticula = An abnormal outpouching of a hollow viscus into the surrounding tissues.

They can be classified by:

- *Aetiology*
  - Congenital (Meckel's diverticulum) versus acquired
  - Pulsion versus traction. Most diverticula are of the pulsion variety. Traction diverticula are much less common and are mostly a consequence of fibrotic healing in lymph nodes secondary to chronic granulomatous disease exerting traction on the neighbouring bowel wall.
- *Location*
  - By site (oesophagus, e.g. Zenker's diverticulum, small intestine, large intestine)
  - Mesenteric (small intestine) versus anti-mesenteric location (Meckel's diverticulum)
- *Architecture*
  - True (Meckel's diverticulum) versus false (sigmoid colon, pharyngeal pouch)

What complications might they undergo?

Complications:

- Perforation
- Inflammation +/– infection
- Bleeding
- Fistulae
- Strictures
- Malignancy (e.g. bladder diverticula)

Thrombosis and emboli

What is the difference between a clot, thrombus and embolus?

A thrombus is defined as 'solid material formed from the constituents of blood in flowing blood' (when formed in stationary blood = clot).

An embolus is defined as 'an abnormal mass of undissolved material that is carried in the bloodstream from one place to another'.

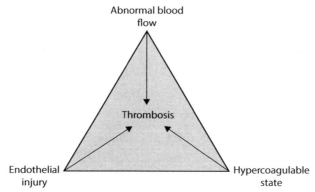

Figure 2.7 Virchow's triad.

What causes a thrombus?

Virchow's triad (see Figure 2.7):

- Damage to vessel wall
- Alterations in blood flow
- Alterations in constituents of blood

What are the different types of emboli?

Can be solid, liquid or gas.

- Thrombus
- Fat
- Air
- Atheromatous material
- Amniotic fluid
- Tumour cells
- Foreign material (e.g. broken cannulae)

Atherosclerosis

What is atherosclerosis? How does it arise? What are the complications?

Atherosclerosis is a chronic inflammatory process.

It is a disease of the tunica intima layer of the vessel wall.

It is reversible upon removing the injurious agent (hence the importance of risk factor modification and primary prevention strategies).

The 'response to injury' hypothesis seems most plausible in terms of explaining the underlying pathogenesis. It explains how the biggest risk factors (namely tobacco toxins, hypertension and turbulent blood flow, lipids and glycosylated haemoglobin in diabetes mellitus) exert their influence and why risk factor modification is so effective in modifying the disease process.

Complications of atherosclerosis include:

- Distal ischaemia
- Vessel occlusion
- Plaque ulceration, rupture
- Thrombosis
- Haemorrhage into a plaque
- Embolism – Lipid or thrombus
- Calcification
- Aneurysm formation

Necrosis and apoptosis

What is necrosis? What are the different types?

Necrosis is abnormal tissue death during life. Necrosis is always pathological and is accompanied by inflammation. Groups of cells are involved and undergo swelling and lysis. Necrotic cells are phagocytosed by inflammatory cells. There are several different types of necrosis:

- Coagulative (structured) necrosis – The most common form of necrosis. Results from interruption of blood supply. Tissue architecture is preserved. Seen in organs supplied by end arteries such as the kidney, heart, liver and spleen.
- Liquefactive (colliquative) necrosis – Occurs in tissues rich in lipid where lysosomal enzymes denature the fat and cause liquefaction of the tissue. Characteristically occurs in the brain.
- Caseous (unstructured) necrosis – Gross appearance is of soft, cheesy friable material. Tissue architecture is destroyed. Commonly seen in TB.
- Fat necrosis – Can occur following direct trauma (e.g. breast) or enzymatic lipolysis (e.g. pancreatitis).
- Fibrinoid necrosis – Seen in the walls of arteries that are subjected to high pressures as in malignant hypertension. The muscular wall undergoes necrosis and is associated with deposition of fibrin.
- Gangrenous necrosis – This is irreversible tissue death characterised by putrefaction. It may be wet, dry or gaseous. The tissues appear green or black because of breakdown of haemoglobin.

What is the difference between apoptosis and necrosis?

Apoptosis	Necrosis
Energy dependent (active)	Energy independent
Internally programmed (suicide)	Response to external injury
Affects single cells	Affects groups of cells
No accompanying inflammation	Accompanied by inflammation
Physiological or pathological	Always pathological
Plasma membrane remains intact	Loss of plasma membrane integrity
Cell shrinkage, fragmentation and formation of apoptotic bodies	Cell swelling and lysis

Hypersensitivity reactions

What is a hypersensitivity reaction? How are they classified?

A hypersensitivity reaction is a condition in which undesirable tissue damage follows the development of humeral or cell mediated immunity. It represents an exaggerated response of the host's immune system to a particular stimulus.

Hypersensitivity reactions can be classified into four classes according to the Gell and Coombs classification. The original description by Gell and Coombs was based on four classes, with a fifth class subsequently being added later.

Gell and Coombs Classification of Hypersensitivity Reactions
Type I – Mast cell degranulation mediated by pre-formed IgE bound to mast cells. Immediate (within minutes). Anaphylaxis, atopic allergies.
Type II – Antibodies directed towards antigens present on the surface of cells or tissue components. Humoral antibodies participate directly in injuring cells by pre-disposing them to phagocytosis or lysis. Good examples are transfusion reactions, autoimmune haemolytic anaemia and Goodpasture's syndrome. Initiates within several hours.
Type III – Formation of antibody–antigen complexes (immune complex mediated). Good examples are the Arthus reaction, serum sickness and systemic lupus erythematosus (SLE). Initiates in several hours.
Type IV – Delayed type of hypersensitivity. Cell mediated. T-lymphocytes involved. Granulomatous conditions. Contact dermatitis. Initiation time is 24–72 hours.
Type V – (more recent addition to the original classification): Due to the formation of stimulatory autoantibodies in autoimmune conditions such as Graves' disease and myasthenia gravis.

Leg ulcers

What is an ulcer? Give some examples of leg ulcers.

An ulcer is a break in an epithelial surface

The commonest leg ulcers are:

- Venous (70% of cases)
- Arterial
- Neuropathic

Other causes include:

- Infections, e.g. TB, leprosy, syphilis
- Malignancy, e.g. squamous cell carcinoma (SCC), basal cell carcinoma (BCC), melanoma, Marjolin's, Kaposi's sarcoma

- Haematological conditions, e.g. haemolytic anaemias, sickle cell, polycythaemia rubra vera, thalassaemia
- Vasculitides, e.g. rheumatoid arthritis, polyarteritis nodosa
- Metabolic, e.g. pyoderma gangrenosum
- Trauma, e.g. lacerations, burns, radiation, self-inflicted
- Iatrogenic, e.g. over-tight bandaging, ill-fitting plaster cast
- Idiopathic

Tumour markers

What is a tumour marker? Give some examples?

A tumour marker is a substance reliably found in the circulation of a patient with neoplasia which is directly related to the presence of the neoplasm, disappears when the neoplasm is treated and reappears when the neoplasm recurs.

Tumour markers may be

- Hormones, e.g. beta-human chorionic gonadotropin (βHCG), calcitonin
- Enzymes, e.g. prostate-specific antigen (PSA), placental alkaline phosphatase (ALP), lactate dehydrogenase (LDH)
- Oncofetal antigens, e.g. α-fetoprotein, carcinoembryonic antigen (CEA), CA-125, CA19-9
- Serum and tissue proteins, e.g. thyroglobulin

What are the possible uses of tumour markers?

- Diagnostic purposes
- Prognostic information (tumour load)
- Monitoring response to treatment
- Surveillance to detect recurrence
- Screening

Colitis

What is colitis? How can it be classified?

Colitis is inflammation of the colon. Colitis can be classified by aetiology into:

- Inflammatory – Ulcerative colitis, Crohn's colitis, indeterminate colitis
- Infective colitis (also includes pseudomembranous colitis caused by *Clostridium difficile* – See Chapter 3)
- Ischaemic colitis
- Radiation colitis
- Collagenous colitis
- Microscopic colitis (and lymphocytic/eosinophilic colitis)

Malignant melanoma

What is malignant melanoma? What are the different types?

Melanoma is a malignant neoplasm of melanocytes.

There are several different subtypes including:

- Superficial spreading (most common, accounting for 70% cases)
- Nodular
- Hutchinson's freckle (lentigo maligna melanoma)
- Acral lentiginous
- Amelanotic

What macroscopic features in naevi are suggestive of melanoma?

Only 10%–20% of melanomas form in pre-existing naevi, with the remainder arising *de novo*. Macroscopic features in a pre-existing naevus that suggest malignant change include:

Asymmetry
Border irregularity
Colour variegation
Diameter >6 mm
Elevation

As well as changes in size, shape and colour, there may also be tingling, itching, crusting, serosanguinous discharge or the presence of satellite lesions.

What are the risk factors for developing melanoma?

Congenital:

- Xeroderma pigmentosum
- Dysplastic naevus syndrome
- BRAF gene mutations (found in up to 80% melanomas)
- Giant congenital pigmented naevus

Acquired:

- Ultraviolet light exposure with a history of sunburn (especially in childhood)
- Past history of melanoma (increases risk three and a half times)
- Red hair
- Tendency to freckle
- Pre-existing skin lesions, e.g. lentigo maligna
- High total number of naevi (>20)
- Immunocomprimised conditions, e.g. HIV, Hodgkin's disease, cyclosporin A therapy

How is malignant melanoma staged?

Breslow's depth is more accurate than Clarke's level because skin thickness varies in different parts of the body.

The Breslow thickness is defined as the tumour invasion depth from the top of the **granular layer** of the epidermis to the deepest point of the tumour.

Stage I – ≤0.75 mm Breslow thickness
Stage II – 0.76–1.50 mm Breslow thickness
Stage III – 1.51–2.25 mm Breslow thickness
Stage IV – 2.26–3.00 mm Breslow thickness
Stage V – >3.00 mm Breslow thickness

Tumour thickness, as defined by the Breslow's depth of invasion, is the most important determinant of prognosis and increased tumour thickness is correlated with a worse prognosis. Thus, 5-year survivals according to Breslow depths are as follows:

<1 mm – 95%–100% 5-year survival
1–2 mm – 80%–96% 5-year survival
2.1–4 mm – 60%–75% 5-year survival
>4 mm – 37%–50% 5-year survival

Tissue diagnosis

What is the difference between cytology and histology?

- Cytology is the study of individual cells and cell morphology. It is usually obtained by fine needle aspiration or brushings from epithelial surfaces.
- Histology studies cells within the context of tissues and provides information about tissue architecture. It is obtained by biopsy.

What are the advantages and disadvantages of each?

Cytology advantages:

- Simple to perform, rapid
- Minimally invasive
- Cheap and requires minimal equipment

Cytology disadvantages:

- Tells you nothing about the tissue architecture. For example, it cannot distinguish a thyroid follicular adenoma from a carcinoma because it cannot assess invasion.
- Large, poorly defined field sampled. This can result in sampling error, or insufficient material for definitive diagnosis. This often results in multiple samples being taken.
- Needs experienced cytologist
- Operator dependent

- Potential for spread of malignant cells
- Less amenable to further studies (e.g. special stains)

Histology advantages:

- Defined lesion sampled
- Provides information on tissue architecture and provides definitive diagnosis of invasion and therefore can aid in the staging of cancers

Histology disadvantages:

- Technically more difficult to perform
- Requires fixation and processing and therefore takes longer to report
- Invasive
- May be painful or distressing to patient
- Expensive
- Potential for spread of malignant cells
- May alter morphology of lesion for subsequent imaging

Referral to the coroner

When would you refer a death to the coroner?

A death should be referred to the HM coroner if:

- The cause of death is unknown
- When a doctor has not attended the deceased within 14 days of death or in terminal illness
- All sudden deaths including all within 24 hours of hospital admission
- The death was violent, unnatural or suspicious
- The death may be due to an accident (whenever it occurred)
- The death may be due to self-neglect or neglect by others
- The death may be due to an industrial disease or related to the deceased's employment
- The death may be due to an abortion
- The death occurred during an operation or before recovery from the effects of an anaesthetic
- The death may be due to suicide
- The death occurred during or shortly after detention in police or prison custody

CHAPTER 3: MICROBIOLOGY

INTRODUCTION TO THE MICROBIOLOGY STATION*

The microbiology station is a relatively recent addition to the Membership of the Royal College of Surgeons (MRCS) Part B objective structured clinical examination (OSCE). Although only one station, this station can often mean the difference

---

* For further reading see *Bailey & Love's Short Practice of Surgery* 27th edition, Chapter 5, 'Surgical infection'

between passing and failing as it is often neglected by many candidates sitting for the exam. It is therefore imperative to prepare well for this station. This chapter covers the common topics that candidates are expected to be familiar with for the exam.

Common topics include the following:

- Gram staining
- Mycobacteria (tuberculosis [TB], as well as atypical mycobacteria)
- Human immunodeficiency virus (HIV)
- Necrotising fasciitis
- Clostridia group of organisms
- Staphylococci, streptococci, methicillin-resistant *Staphylococcus aureus* (MRSA)
- Pseudomonas
- Infective endocarditis (including Duke's criteria)
- Taking blood cultures

BACTERIA – CLASSIFICATION, GRAM STAINING AND SEPSIS

How do we classify bacteria and give examples?

Bacteria can be classified according to their

- Staining properties – Gram-positive, Gram-negative, acid-fast etc.
- Morphology – Round (cocci), rods (bacilli), spiral (spirochaetes), comma-shaped (vibrio), flagellated, possession of a capsule etc.
- Oxygen requirements – Aerobic or anaerobic; obligate or facultative
- Ability to form spores – Spore-forming or non-spore forming

In **Gram-positive** bacteria, the peptidoglycan forms a thick (20–80 nm) layer external to the cell membrane. In **Gram-negative** species, the peptidoglycan layer is thinner (only 5–10 nm) but is overlaid by an outer membrane. The principal molecules in the outer membrane of Gram-negative bacteria are lipopolysaccharides.

These structural differences form the basis of the Gram stain. Gram-positive bacteria are able to retain an iodine purple dye complex when exposed to a brief alcohol wash. Gram-negative bacteria have a smaller cell wall but a higher lipid content and as a result the alcohol washes away the purple dye. Gram-positive bacteria appear **blue** and Gram-negative bacteria are counterstained with a **pink** dye.

As a tip for the examination:

- All cocci are Gram-positive (except Neisseria which causes meningitis and gonorrhoea)
- All bacilli are Gram-negative (except Clostridia, Mycobacteria and the organisms that cause anthrax, listeria, diphtheria and actinomycosis)

What is the 'Sepsis Six'?

The 'Sepsis Six' is a series of three diagnostic and three therapeutic steps (all to be delivered within 1 hour of the initial diagnosis of sepsis) designed to reduce the mortality associated with sepsis. It was designed in 2006 as part of the 'Surviving Sepsis Campaign' and its use has been associated with a reduction in mortality, decreased length of hospital stay and fewer Intensive Treatment Unit (ITU) admissions.

1. Deliver high-flow oxygen

2. Take blood cultures

3. Administer empiric intravenous (IV) antibiotics

4. Measure serum lactate and full blood count (FBC)

5. Start IV fluid resuscitation

6. Commence measurement of accurate urine output

STAPHYLOCOCCI AND STREPTOCOCCI

What properties do staphylococci exhibit?

Staphylococci are Gram-positive cocci and form 'grape-like' clusters. They are catalase positive (unlike streptococci and enterococci which are catalase negative).

They can be classified into coagulase positive organisms (e.g. *S. aureus*) and coagulase negative microbes (e.g. *Streptococcus epidermidis*).

S. aureus causes a diverse array of infections and is a common cause of skin infections (e.g. cellulitis), food poisoning, infective endocarditis, septic arthritis and osteomyelitis (Figures 3.1 and 3.2).

What is special about MRSA?

MRSA is resistant to beta-lactam antibiotics which includes the penicillins and cephalosporins. This resistance makes the infection more difficult to treat with standard antibiotics often resulting in a more severe form of infection requiring vancomycin.

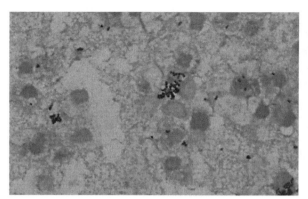

Figure 3.1 Staphylococcal pus.

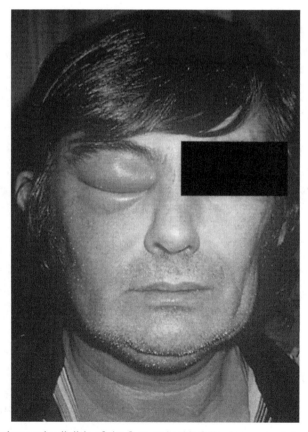

Figure 3.2 Staphylococcal cellulitis of the face and orbit following severe infection of an epidermoid cyst of the scalp.

What other resistant organisms are you aware of other than MRSA?

VRE = vancomycin resistant Enterococci

CPE = carbapenem-resistant Enterobacteriaceae

Why and how is screening for MRSA performed?

Screening for MRSA is performed in all the National Health Service (NHS) surgical patients (one-third of individuals are colonised at any one time with *S. aureus* and around 3% are colonised with MRSA). MRSA screening helps to reduce the chance of patients developing an MRSA infection or passing an infection on to other vulnerable patients. Most hospital trusts have a topical decolonisation protocol which usually involves a 5-day course of mupirocin nasal ointment T.D.S. to both nostrils and chlorhexidine 4% body wash daily for 5 days. Complete eradication is not always possible but a decrease in carriage may reduce the risk of transmission in health-care settings and reduce the risk of inoculation to the patient's own surgical wound during surgery. For MRSA carriers, ideally elective surgery should be scheduled for day 5 of decolonisation.

What properties do streptococci exhibit?

- Gram-positive cocci that form chains
- Catalase negative
- Classified by haemolytic patterns (alpha-, beta-, gamma-) and beta-haemolytic bacteria further classified by Lancefield antigen groups

What infections do Streptococcus pyogenes cause?

Group A streptococci (= *S. pyogenes*) are responsible for causing acute bacterial tonsillitis, skin infections (impetigo/cellulitis), scarlet fever, necrotising fasciitis, rheumatic fever and post-streptococcal glomerulonephritis, amongst others (Figures 3.3 and 3.4).

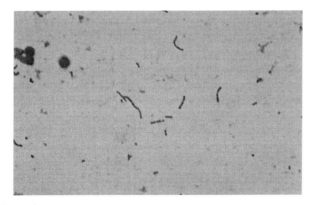

Figure 3.3 Streptococci.

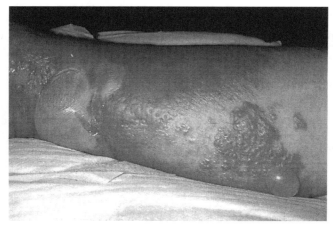

Figure 3.4 Streptococcal cellulitis of the leg following a minor puncture wound.

MYCOBACTERIA

What are mycobacteria?

- Mycobacteria are obligate aerobic, rod-shaped, non-spore forming, non-motile bacilli with a waxy coat that causes them to retain certain stains after being treated with acid and alcohol; they are therefore known as *acid–alcohol-fast bacilli* (AAFB).
- Mycobacteria do not readily take up the Gram stain but they would be Gram-positive if the Gram stain could penetrate their waxy walls.

How are they classified?

Typical mycobacteria – *Mycobacterium tuberculosis, Mycobacterium bovis, Mycobacterium leprae*

Atypical mycobacteria (also known as *non-tuberculous mycobacteria*) – An important, diverse class of microorganisms that is commonly resistant to standard anti-tuberculous medications and exhibit different characteristics and growth rates in culture. Examples include *Mycobacterium avium intracellulare, Mycobacterium kansasii, Mycobacterium malmoense* to name just a few examples. They are responsible for causing lymphadenopathy in paediatric patients (particularly in the head and neck region) and in immunosuppressed individuals.

How are mycobacteria detected?

- The Ziehl–Neelsen stain is used instead to visualise the organisms, which stain pinkish red.

- Polymerase chain reaction.
- Interferon gamma assays (e.g. Quantiferon).
- They can be cultured in Löwenstein–Jensen medium. This may take up to 6 weeks.

How are they treated?

TB – Standard regimens consist of 'RIPE' treatment (rifampicin, isoniazid, pyrazinamide, ethambutol). Six months of treatment are required.

Non-tuberculous mycobacteria – May be treated either with surgical excision (lymphadenectomy) or prolonged courses of antibiotics (e.g. clarithromycin, rifampicin, ethambutol). Incision and drainage is contraindicated as it may lead to a chronically discharging sinus.

CLOSTRIDIA

This is a hot exam topic.

What properties do the Clostridia family of bacteria share?

All members of the *Clostridia* group of organisms have the following properties:

- Gram-positive bacilli
- Obligate anaerobes
- Spore-forming
- Saprophytic (i.e. live in the soil)
- Motile (but non-invasive)
- Exotoxin-producing (Figure 3.5)

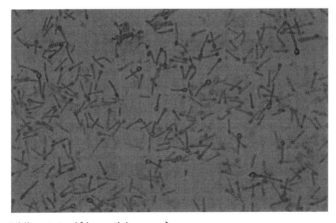

Figure 3.5 *Clostridium tetani* (drumstick spores).

Name some members of the family that are important in surgery?

Clostridia are responsible for causing several diseases in man

- *Clostridium tetani* (responsible for causing tetanus)
- *Clostridium botulinum* (responsible for causing botulism and the toxin can be harvested as 'Botox' and utilised in surgery)
- *Clostridium perfringens*, formerly known as *Clostridium welchii* (responsible for causing gas gangrene and food poisoning)
- *Clostridium difficile* (responsible for causing pseudomembranous colitis, also known as antibiotic-associated diarrhoea)

How does 'Botox' work and name some uses of botulinum toxin in surgery?

Botulinum toxin ('Botox') is taken up into pre-synaptic terminals of nerve endings and prevents release of acetylcholine, thereby paralysing muscles and prevents parasympathetic nerve transmission. Uses in surgery include:

- Anal fissures
- Treatment of achalasia
- Treatment of Frey's syndrome (gustatory sweating) or a salivary leak following parotid surgery
- Treatment of cricopharyngeal spasm
- Treatment of spasmodic dysphonia
- Management of hypertonic speech following laryngectomy
- Hyperhidrosis
- Dystonias, e.g. blepharospasm
- Cosmesis

Botox is contraindicated in myasthenia gravis.

NECROTISING FASCIITIS

What is necrotising fasciitis?

Necrotising fasciitis is a rapidly progressive inflammatory infection of the fascia, with secondary necrosis of the subcutaneous tissues. Necrotising fasciitis moves along the fascial planes.

'Fournier gangrene' is a form of necrotising fasciitis that is localised to the scrotum and perineal area.

What microbes are commonly responsible for causing necrotising fasciitis?

In necrotising fasciitis, group A haemolytic streptococci and *S. aureus*, alone or in synergism, are frequently the initiating infecting bacteria. However, other aerobic and anaerobic pathogens may be present, including the following:

Bacteroides, Clostridium, Peptostreptococcus, Enterobacteriaceae, Coliforms
(e.g. *Escherichia coli*), *Proteus, Pseudomonas, Klebsiella*

How is it treated?

- Always start with resuscitation, including ABCDE (Airway, Breathing, Circulation, Disability, Exposure)
- Wound debridement
- High-dose intravenous antibiotics
- Hyperbaric oxygen
- *Interdisciplinary* team approach (plastic surgeons, intensivists, microbiologists, wound care nurses etc.) (Figure 3.6)

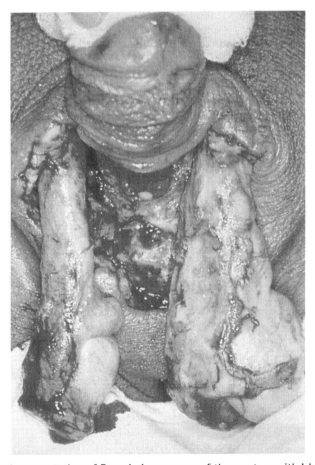

Figure 3.6 A classic presentation of Fournier's gangrene of the scrotum with 'shameful exposure of the testes' following excision of the gangrenous skin.

TRANSMISSION AND PREVENTION OF INFECTIONS IN THE OPERATING THEATRE INCLUDING HIV

What precautions should be taken in operating theatres to avoid infections?

Design of theatre suites:

- Theatre sited away from main hospital traffic
- Clear designated areas of asepsis
- Vents kept open, doors closed

Appropriate ventilation:

- Positive pressure ventilation (20 air changes per hour)
- Laminar airflow systems (300 air changes per hour)

Theatre staff:

- Minimum number of individuals, avoidance of excess traffic
  Operating personnel

- Aseptic technique – Hand decontamination, sterile gowns, gloves, caps, masks
  Patient preparation

- Optimise patient nutritional status, minimal pre-op hospital stay, pre-op showering, hair removal at time of surgery (rather than prior to surgery), identification of MRSA carriers, prophylactic antibiotics, role of mechanical bowel preparation controversial

Skin preparation:

- Iodine or chlorhexidine, sterile wound drapes, sterile equipment

Surgical technique:

- Speed, minimising spillage, meticulous haemostasis, avoiding dead space, avoidance of unwarranted drains, minimising foreign material, wound irrigation, choice of suture/closure material (infection rates [IRs] – braided > monofilament; sutures > clips > steristrips), autoclaving instruments

- The National Institute for Health and Clinical Excellence (NICE) has produced guidance on the prevention and treatment of surgical site infection and it is worth being familiar with these prior to the exam.

What precautions would you take as a surgeon when operating on a known HIV positive patient?

When operating on a patient whom is known, or suspected, to have an infectious condition, universal precautions should be taken in the usual manner (these are the precautions taken to protect theatre staff from infection with all cases, i.e. every patient is treated as if they are infected), plus additional, special precautions should be taken

Pre-operatively:

- Inform anaesthetist and theatre staff about high-risk patient
- Maximal use of disposable instruments
- Put the patient last on the theatre list (unlike diabetic patients and those with latex allergy who should go first)
- Consider appropriate antibiotic prophylaxis

Intra-operatively:

- Use an apron, boots rather than shoes, gown, cap, mask, face visors (eye protection)
- Cover up non-intact skin surfaces
- Consider double gloving and use of 'indicator' glove systems
- Ensure good haemostasis throughout
- Use diathermy rather than a scalpel
- Ensure sharps are discarded quickly and efficiently, with no hand-to-hand passage of sharps, a 'no-touch' surgical technique when handling needles, no handheld needles, use of blunt needles where possible and avoiding resheathing of needles
- Ensure theatre staff and equipment are kept to a minimum
- Ensure spills are cleaned up meticulously
- Pathology should be notified in advance of infectious specimens and all infectious specimens labelled as high risk

Post-operatively:

- Patients are at high risk of wound infections, dehiscence and delayed healing

Special precautions are also used for infective cases to prevent spread of infection to other patients, e.g. MRSA, Acinetobacter etc.

How may surgical wounds be classified?

- *Clean* – An incision in which no inflammation is encountered in a surgical procedure, without a break in sterile technique, and during which the respiratory, alimentary or genitourinary tracts are not entered (e.g. thyroidectomy). Infection rate (IR) = 1.5%–5.1%

- *Clean-contaminated* – An incision through which the respiratory, alimentary or genitourinary tract is entered under controlled conditions but with no contamination encountered (e.g. cholecystectomy). IR = 7.7%–10.8%
- *Contaminated* – An incision undertaken during an operation in which there is a major break in sterile technique or gross spillage from the gastrointestinal tract, or an incision in which acute, non-purulent inflammation is encountered. Open traumatic wounds that are more than 12–24 hours old also fall into this category (e.g. elective colorectal surgery). IR = 15.2%–16.3%
- *Dirty or infected* – An incision undertaken during an operation in which the viscera are perforated or when acute inflammation with pus is encountered, and for traumatic wounds where treatment is delayed, there is faecal contamination or devitalised tissue is present (e.g. emergency surgery for faecal peritonitis from a colonic perforation). IR = 28.0%–40.0%

When are prophylactic antibiotics indicated in surgery?

As per the NICE guidelines on surgical site infection, antibiotic prophylaxis should be given to patients before

- Clean surgery involving the placement of a graft, implant or prosthesis
- Clean-contaminated surgery
- Contaminated surgery

Avoid using antibiotic prophylaxis routinely for clean non-prosthetic uncomplicated surgery unless an infection would be very severe or have life-threatening consequences.

In the United Kingdom, NICE no longer recommend antibiotic prophylaxis in patients with valvular heart disease at risk of infective endocarditis because there is limited clinical evidence of its effectiveness and there are negative effects of taking antibiotics that may outweigh the benefits (e.g. allergic reactions and increased bacterial resistance).

INFECTIVE ENDOCARDITIS

A patient with a fever and a *new* heart murmur is infective endocarditis until proven otherwise.

What are the risk factors for infective endocarditis?

Damaged heart valves (e.g. rheumatic fever), prosthetic valves, intravenous drug users (IVDUs), poor dentition, immunosuppression.

What microorganisms are responsible for causing endocarditis?

- Viridans streptococci commonly
- *S. aureus* (in IVDUs, classically causing right-sided endocarditis and affecting the tricuspid valve)
- *S. epidermidis* (commonly affecting prosthetic valves)
- *Streptococcus bovis* (associated with colonic malignancies)
- HACEK group of microorganisms – *Haemophilus, Actinobacillus, Cardiobacterium, Eikinella, Kingella*
- Fungi and yeasts (e.g. Candida and Aspergillus)

How is infective endocarditis diagnosed?

Duke criteria. Definitive diagnosis requires two major criteria, one major and three minor criteria or five minor criteria.

Major criteria	Minor criteria
1. Two separate positive blood cultures with typical microorganisms that cause endocarditis	2. Fever > 38.0°C
3. Evidence of endocardial involvement with a positive echocardiogram (e.g. vegetations, abscess, prosthetic heart valve dehiscence, new valvular regurgitation)	4. Predisposing factors – known cardiac lesions, IVDUs
	5. Embolic phenomena – arterial emboli, pulmonary infarcts, Janeway lesions
	6. Immunological phenomena – Osler's nodes, Roth spots, glomerulonephritis, rheumatoid factor
	7. Microbiological evidence – positive blood cultures not meeting major criteria or serological evidence of infection

What are the causes of culture-negative endocarditis?

- Recent antibiotics (commonest cause)
- Difficult to culture organisms – *Coxiella, Chlamydia, Bartonella, Gemella*
- Non-bacterial organisms – Candida, fungi
- Slow-growing microorganisms with fastidious growth requirements – HACEK group

- Connective tissue diseases – Libman–Sacks, marantic endocarditis
- Wrong/alternative diagnosis, e.g. atrial myxoma not infective endocarditis vegetation
- Penetrated organisms – Aortic root abscess, septic emboli etc.
- Poor culture techniques, sampling error – Cultures taken in abacteraemic phase
- Right-sided endocarditis

How is infective endocarditis treated?

High-dose IV antibiotics for 2–6 weeks duration. The exact regimen and doses will be dictated by local microbiological guidelines and microbiology advice should be sought early.

What are the indications for surgical debridement in infective endocarditis?

- Significant valvular disease
- Haemodynamic compromise
- Intracardiac complications – Abscess, conductive defects, destructive lesions
- Fungal infection
- Resistant organisms
- Recurrent septic emboli despite high-dose IV antibiotics
- Persistent positive blood cultures despite appropriate antibiotics
- Prosthetic valve dehiscence
- Relapsing infection in presence of prosthetic valve

TAKING BLOOD CULTURES

What are the indications for taking blood cultures?

Indications for blood culture:

- Pyrexia of unknown origin (PUO)
- To identify subacute bacteraemia (e.g. subacute bacterial endocarditis)

Describe the steps in taking blood cultures.

You may be asked to demonstrate this in the exam and you must be well prepared for this. The steps are as follows:

Introduction:

1. Blood cultures are best taken when the patient spikes a fever (maximal bacteraemia).

2. Introduce yourself to the patient, check patient's identity, explain procedure, confirm indication and gain informed consent.

Positioning:

3. Ensure that the patient is comfortable (e.g. lying or sitting position).

4. Support the arm from which blood is to be taken with a pillow.

Procedure:

5. Gather relevant equipment – Pair of culture bottles (aerobic and anaerobic), needle, 20 mL syringe, Vacutainer system, tourniquet, sterile gloves of appropriate size, alcohol wipe/Betadine etc.

6. Aseptic technique at all times.

7. Wash hands and put on sterile gloves.

8. Clean the entrance ports of the blood culture bottles with an alcohol wipe and allow to dry for at least 30 seconds.

9. Apply a tourniquet proximal to the elbow crease, and palpate for and select a vein.

10. Clean the skin (venepuncture site) with an alcohol wipe/Betadine and wait approximately 30 seconds for the alcohol to evaporate (do not take blood cultures via an existing IV cannula).

11. Do not re-palpate the venepuncture site once it has been cleaned.

12. With a conventional needle/syringe, the anaerobic bottle is filled first to avoid introducing air into anaerobic bottle (N.B. air rises). N.B. If the winged butterfly needle technique is used, air is present in the line and therefore the aerobic bottle is best filled first.

13. Although it used to be advised to change needles before filling the first bottle and between bottles in order to reduce the risk of contamination, this is no longer advised as it increases the risk of needle-stick injuries.

14. At least 10 mL of blood should be placed into each bottle.

15. Remove the tourniquet, apply pressure over the venepuncture site and withdraw the needle.

16. Gain haemostasis from the venepuncture site by applying cotton wool until bleeding has stopped and dispose of all sharps safely in a sharps bin.

17. Label both bottles at the bedside. Label the blood cultures with the patient's details (name, date of birth and hospital number) and the date and time when the blood sample was taken.

18. Complete the relevant microbiology investigation request form, stating the test required (MC&S – microscopy and culture), the indication for the test, the clinical details, the site from which the sample was taken and whether the patient is taking any antibiotics.

19. Wash your hands or use alcohol gel.

20. Try to gather three sets of blood cultures separated in time and space (especially for endocarditis) to improve the sensitivity.

21. Start empirical antibiotics after cultures taken to avoid culture-negative (false negative) results.

Important points:

- Blood cultures should be performed prior to commencing antibiotics.
- Each set of blood cultures consists of an anaerobic and aerobic blood culture bottle.
- A fever occurs between 30 and 120 minutes after the introduction of bacteria into the circulation.
- Ideally, three sets of blood cultures should be performed from at least two different sites.
- If a central line is in situ, blood cultures should be sent from blood taken from the line.

CHAPTER 4: APPLIED SURGICAL SCIENCE

Human immunodeficiency virus in surgery

Venous thromboembolism

Monitoring during anaesthesia

Post-operative complications

Blood transfusions

Day case surgery

The multiply injured patient: Advanced trauma life support – Principles and practice

OPERATING ROOM*

How would you construct and organise the ideal operating room?

- Location – Near the Intensive Care, Accident and Emergency and Radiology Departments.
- Separate from the general hospital traffic.
- A single floor should be reserved for the operating suites.
- Reduce solar heat gain or loss; the operating suites should be located in the lower hospital levels.
- Streams of clean and dirty traffic should be separated to avoid contamination.
- There should be a transfer and changeover area at the entry and exit points.
- There should be protective areas – Recovery, changing room and offices.
- There should be at least three zones – Clean, sterile and disposal.
  - *Clean zone* – Scrub rooms, gowning areas, exit lobby, rest areas and sterile stores
  - *Sterile zone* – The operating theatre and sterile preparation rooms
  - *Disposal zone* – The least clean area: Disposal sluice or sink rooms
- Hospital staff should move from one clean area to another without having to pass through unprotected or traffic areas.
- Airflow direction should be from the clean to less clean areas. There should be no airflow between theatre suites.
- Heating, air-conditioning and ventilation should allow for comfortable working conditions.
- The operating suites should have good lighting (artificial and natural).
  - General lightening of theatres should be provided by fluorescent tubes or filament lamps producing illumination with little or no glaze.
  - The main operating lights are compared by direct light from several angles to reduce shadows.
- Electricity should be maintained with emergency support (supplementary generator) in case of power failure. The main voltage is between 220 and 240 V, 50 Hz AC. Switches and sockets should be spark-free.

---

* For further reading, see *Bailey and Love's Short Practice of Surgery* 27th edition, Chapter 18, 'Anaesthesia and Pain Relief'

- A clean environment is important.
  - Smooth surfaces that are easily washable.
  - Joins between walls, ceiling and floors should be curved to reduce dirty collection.
  - The floors should be impervious with anti-static properties. They should be easy to wash and may be comprised of rubber or vinyl.
- The colour of the operating suites should be pale-blue, grey or green in order to be less tiring on the eyes.

In the operating theatre, what is the goal of ventilation?

The main goals of ventilation are as follows:

- Comfort to all hospital staff
- Removal of anaesthetic gas
- Admit air that is free of pathological organisms

What types of ventilation are used in operating rooms?

The aim of the airflow system is to prevent airborne microorganisms entering the surgical wound. Ventilation should allow air to pass through a steam humidifier, resulting in 50%–60% relative humidity. Combined with background heating, the ventilation system can be used to adjust the temperature in the operating suites to between 18.5° and 22°C. After filteration, air is introduced at ceiling height and exhausted near the floor with at least 20 air changes per hour. The operating theatre is maintained at a positive pressure relative to the surroundings.

Turbulent air flow system

Positive pressure is used to prevent dirty air entering the sterile operating suites. The air pressure should be higher than the surrounding areas. Air is drawn by fans via filters and humidified into the operating areas.

Laminar flow displacement system

The high impact and high exhaust system was first introduced by Charnley. Airflow moves at a unidirectional horizontal velocity and passes through filters to remove contamination. Positive pressurisation is used. The displaced air in not recycled but moves away from the operating site. Laminar airflow provides 100-300 air changes per hour and is used in cases involving insertion of implants (e.g. joint replacements) to avoid airborne infection.

SAFETY IN THE OPERATING THEATRE*

Patient safety is paramount, both inside and outside the operating theatre. A surgeon must always make patient safety and well-being their number one priority.

---

* For further reading, see *Bailey and Love's Short Practice of Surgery,* 27th edition, Chapter 20, 'Postoperative care'.

This not only applies within the operating theatre, but also before and after any operation, when the patient is just as vulnerable. As medical students, we are always taught the old aphorism *primum non nocere* (which as you may recall means 'first do no harm') and you must never forget this, as you advance and progress in your chosen specialty. Ultimately, the surgeon is responsible for any patient that is under his or her care.

Adequate preventative measures should always be put in place to ensure that the risks posed to hospital patients are kept to an absolute minimum. However, incidents do occasionally occur and it is always a good practice to report any 'near misses' or actual incidents to the appropriate authority at the earliest opportunity. This may be done at a local level by completing an incident form, which is then dealt with by the trust risk management team, as part of the hospital Clinical Governance Committee. At a national level, incidents can be reported directly to the National Patient Safety Agency, whose responsibility is to collect, analyse and audit such data on a national scale and suggest and implement changes to improve patient safety. It is worth mentioning this as part of any answer to a question that touches on patient safety for bonus marks!

How should the surgeon ensure the patient's safety in theatre?

- Surgical safety checklist – In 2008, the World Health Organisation (WHO) published guidelines of recommended practices to reduce the rate of preventable surgical complications and deaths worldwide. A set of checks has been incorporated into the WHO surgical safety checklist, which is completed for every patient undergoing a surgical procedure. In the United Kingdom, a five-step process is used to improve theatre communication and to verify and check the surgical procedure (Figure 4.1).

WHO Surgical Safety Checklist: UK process

- Step 1 – Pre-list briefing
- Step 2 – Sign in
- Step 3 – Time out
- Step 4 – Sign out
- Step 5 – Post-list debriefing

- Check the patient's details to ensure the correct patient has been consented for the correct procedure
- Check the patient has been marked correctly
- Ensure the patient is suitably prepared
  - Suitably starved
  - Consented
  - Appropriate antibiotics prescribed and given
  - Deep vein thrombosis (DVT) prophylaxis

Surgical safety checklist (first edition)

Before induction of anaesthesia

Sign In

☐ Patient has confirmed
  • Identity
  • Site
  • Procedure
  • Consent

☐ Site marked/not applicable

☐ Anaesthesia safety check completed

☐ Pulse oximeter on patient and fuctioning

Does patient have a:

Known allergy?
☐ No
☐ Yes

Difficult airway/aspiration risk?
☐ No
☐ Yes, and equipment/assistance available

Risk of >500 mL blood loss
(7 mL/kg in children)?
☐ No
☐ Yes, and adequate intravenous access
  and fluids planned

Before skin incision

Time Out

☐ Confirm all team members have
  introduced themselves by name
  and role

☐ Surgeon, anaesthesia professional
  and nurse verbally confirm
  • Patient
  • Site
  • Procedure

☐ Anticipated critical events

☐ Surgeon reviews: what are the
  critical or unexpected steps,
  operative duration, anticipated
  blood loss?

☐ Anaesthesia team reviews: are there
  any patient-specific concerns?

☐ Nursing team reviews: has sterility
  (including indicator results) been
  confirmed? are there equipment
  issues or any concerns?

Has antibiotic prophylaxis been given
within the last 60 minutes?
☐ Yes
☐ Not applicable

Is essential imaging displayed?
☐ Yes
☐ Not applicable

Before patient leaves operating room

Sign Out

☐ Nurse verbally confirms with the team:

☐ The name of the procedure recorded

☐ That instrument, sponge and needle
  counts are correct (or not applicable)

☐ How the specimen is labelled
  (including patient name)

☐ Whether there are any equipment
  problems to be addressed

☐ Surgeon, anaesthesia professional
  and nurse review the key concerns
  for recovery and management
  of this patient

Figure 4.1 WHO surgical safety checklist.

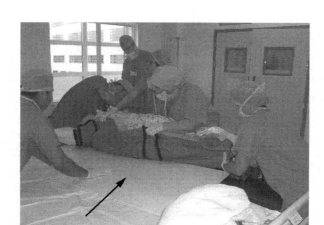

Figure 4.2 Patient transfer. Enough personnel are available to undertake the transfer. The anaesthetist supervises and protects the head, neck and airway. The patient is rolled and a sliding board (arrow) is placed under the patient and undersheet or canvas, which will allow the patient to slide across to the bed in a controlled fashion. Care is being taken by all of the team members to protect the whole patient.

- Safe transfer (Figure 4.2)
  - The patient's transfer is coordinated by the anaesthetist, who protects the airway and connections during the transfer.
- Positioning of the patient and prevention of nerve and pressure injuries
- Eyelids taped to protect the corneas
- Ensure equipment is available and functioning correctly prior to carrying out the procedure
- Aseptic technique throughout, with universal precautions (Figure 4.3)
- Correct and safe use of diathermy and lasers – This is the surgeon's responsibility
- Apply tourniquets correctly with the appropriate time of starting noted
- Check name, dose and expiry date of any medications given intra-operatively Check whether the patient has any known allergies
- Ensure the swab counts are correct at the beginning and end of the operation

What would you do at the end of an operation if the nurse informs you that the final swab count is incorrect?

- Check the initial swab count was correct
- Ask the nursing staff to re-count
- If there is still a discrepancy, inform the theatre coordinator in charge of theatres so that extra support can be provided
- Inform the senior surgeon responsible for the patient
- Inform the anaesthetist about the reason for the delay and ask him or her to kindly keep the patient asleep until the situation has been resolved

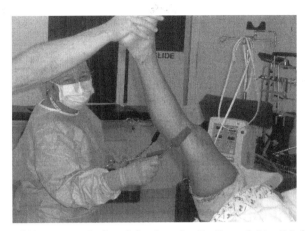

Figure 4.3 Prepping (skin preparation) and draping. Application of skin disinfectant solution to skin. Note that this is the second coat being applied to the posterior aspect of the leg. The leg holder is standing away from the scrub nurse and should be gloved. For this operation, the foot is not being prepped.

- No item including clinical waste must be removed from the theatre
- Perform a thorough search until the missing swabs are found:
  - Commence with a thorough search of the operative area, including all drapes and trolleys
  - Then extend the search to the operating theatre (including the anaesthetic area)
  - Check there are no swabs on the floor or around the patient
  - Search for discarded swabs in the rubbish and laundry bags
- If all the above fails, an x-ray should be taken before the patient leaves the operating theatre, whilst still under anaesthetic. The x-ray must be visibly examined by the surgeon in charge.
- If necessary re-open and explore the wound
- Once the discrepancy has been rectified, a full swab count must be undertaken again and the surgeon informed audibly
- Document the events in the patient's notes and the theatre register
- Complete an incident form and inform the clinical risk manager immediately

How would you manage anaphylaxis in theatre secondary to a drug or latex allergy?

Management of anaphylaxis includes discontinuation of the exposure (e.g. latex) and should follow the usual guidelines for managing anaphylaxis in general. It includes management of the airway, breathing, circulation and administration of resuscitation drugs, with the support of the anaesthetic staff. Adrenaline (epinephrine) is the single most important drug and should be administered intramuscularly (IM). Repeat injections or infusions may be necessary. Other drugs include intravenous (IV) fluids, antihistamines, bronchodilators and corticosteroids. Document in the notes and complete an incident form.

How will you prepare a patient with a known latex allergy for theatre?

There is currently no cure for latex allergy and avoidance of latex containing products is the best way to reduce the risk.

- Identification of high-risk groups – Try to determine whether latex causes an irritant contact dermatitis (non-immune), an allergic contact dermatitis (delayed, type IV hypersensitivity reaction) or full-blown anaphylaxis (type 1 hypersensitivity reaction).
- Providing a latex free environment – All the anaesthetic and surgical equipment containing latex (e.g. gloves) should be replaced with latex free alternatives.
- The patient's identity band, notes and drug chart should state latex allergy.
- Close coordination between all the health-care personnel involved in the patient's care to ensure that wherever possible the patient is scheduled as the **first** case of the day when the airborne latex particles will be at a minimum.
- The theatre should be identified as treating a patient with latex allergy to avoid other staff entering with latex gloves, or others entering without washing their hands after taking off latex gloves.
- Ensure all IV equipment is latex free.
- Every hospital should have a protocol in place for managing such patients and a latex free trolley should be readily available.

How are patient outcomes and deaths audited?

Through the National Confidential Enquiry into Patient Outcome and Deaths (NCEPOD), a national body whose aim is to review clinical practice and identify potentially remediable factors in the practice of anaesthesia, surgery and other invasive medical procedures. NCEPOD reports annually on a particular facet of surgical care and makes recommendations for practice.

PATIENT POSITIONING*

Why is correct patient positioning so important?

It is important to enable adequate access to the operation site and to prevent the patient sliding off the operating table. Side supports may be needed if the patient is being placed into a semi-decubitus lateral position. It is also important to avoid injuries to the patient.

Nerve injuries

Most are due to careless positioning of the patient and inadequate padding resulting in direct compression. They can also result from direct surgical injury, compression

---

* For further reading, see *Bailey and Love's Short Practice of Surgery 27th edition,* Chapter 20, 'Postoperative care'.

by tourniquets, traction and ischaemia secondary to hypotension. They are most likely to occur in extreme positions and prolonged surgery.

Most are due to a neurapraxia. Ninety percent undergo complete recovery; 10% are left with residual weakness or sensory loss.

Pressure sores

The operating table will be padded but additional soft padding under the occiput (horseshoe head support), back, buttocks, elbows and heels (heel protectors) may be required dependent on the patient's position for surgery.

Predisposing factors include elderly, malnourished, excessively thin or obese patients, patients on steroids or those with peripheral vascular disease.

Joint injuries (fractures and dislocations)

Inappropriate handling and positioning may aggravate spinal or joint disorders. Special care is needed in patients with prosthetic hip joints.

Joints are most at risk in the lithotomy position and where there is a 'break' in the operating table. Be alert to the possibility of atlanto-axial dislocation in rheumatoid arthritis patients.

Diathermy burns

No part of the skin surface should be in any contact with any metal if diathermy is being used.

Muscle injury

Compartment syndrome may occur after prolonged surgery, e.g. lithotomy position.

Eye injuries

Eyes should be closed and taped to prevent injury.

Deep vein thrombosis

Poor patient positioning during prolonged surgery increases the risk of DVTs.

Name some common nerve injuries due to incorrect patient positioning.

Ulnar nerve:

- Caused by arms held beside the patient in pronation
- Ulnar nerve compressed at the elbow between the table and medial epicondyle
- Prevented by positioning the arms in supination, with additional padding to protect the ulnar nerve at the elbow

Brachial plexus:

- Caused by excessive arm abduction or external rotation
- Prevented by avoiding more than 60° abduction and preventing the arm from falling off the side of the table

Common peroneal nerve:

- Caused by direct pressure on the nerve with the legs in the lithotomy position
- Nerve compressed against the neck of the fibula
- Prevented by adequate padding of lithotomy poles

Radial nerve:

- Caused by compression from the operating table or arm board
- Also caused by tourniquets or misplaced injections in the deltoid muscle
- Prevented by adequate padding of tourniquets

Eyes and optic nerve:

- Direct pressure from surgical instruments and elbows resting over face

---

Pressure areas which must be given special consideration

- The skin over bony prominences
- Nerves in superficial courses, e.g. common peroneal nerve (take care with placement of the calves in leg supports)
- Nerves at risk of stretch injury, e.g. brachial plexus (head should be neutral where possible)
- Areas at risk of developing a compartment syndrome
- Eye protection – Eyes should be protected from direct pressure (particularly in the prone position), corneal abrasion and splash injuries. Ointment, or eye closure with tape and/or eye pads may be used.

TOURNIQUETS

What are the indications and uses of tourniquets?

Tourniquets are commonly used in surgical practice. When properly used they:

- Provide excellent haemostasis
- Prevent systemic toxicity in isolated limb perfusion techniques and regional IV anaesthesia (Bier's block)

When incorrectly used they are dangerous. Cuff failure can be disastrous with rapid systemic absorption of drugs (e.g. local anaesthetics)

What safeguards should the surgeon take when using tourniquets?

- Note the distal neurovascular status before application
- Ensure correct placement and connection

- Use adequate padding to prevent pressure necrosis
- Exsanguinate the limb before inflation
- Use minimal pressure – Usually 100 mmHg above systolic blood pressure (BP)
- Use for minimal duration – No longer than 90 minutes
- Avoid multiple inflations or deflations
- Check return of circulation and sensation after deflation

What are the contraindications to using a tourniquet?

- Peripheral vascular disease
- In patients at high risk for venous thrombosis (previous DVT or pulmonary embolism [PE])
- Vasculitic disorders
- Sickle cell anaemia

What are the complications of tourniquets?

At the tourniquet site:

- Skin – Friction burns, chemical burns
- Nerve injury
- Increased post-operative pain

Distal to the tourniquet:

- Vascular – Injury/thrombosis
- Muscular – Ischaemia and reperfusion injury. Possible compartment syndrome

Systemic:

- Post-tourniquet syndrome (haemodynamic changes; ↓TPR)
- Post-operative embolic events (hypercoagulability)
- Myoglobinuria
- Increased blood viscosity
- Hypercapnoea and metabolic changes – Elevated potassium and lactate from involved limb after deflation

---

Application of tourniquet

- Appropriate size should be selected
- Apply as proximally as possible
- Apply padding to site without creases
- Apply tightly enough to avoid slippage, but not so tightly as to impede exsanguination
- Exsanguinate the limb prior to inflating the tourniquet using elevation, an Esmarch bandage or a roll cylinder
- When the tourniquet is inflated, the time must be noted
- When the tourniquet is removed, the site should be inspected for damage and the limb for return of circulation. This should be recorded in the notes (with the time)

STETHOSCOPE IN SURGERY

What are the uses of the stethoscope in surgery?

Pre-operative

Assessment of organ systems:
- Cardiovascular conditions (e.g. murmurs)
- Blood pressure measurement
- Vascular conditions (e.g. carotid and renal bruits, ankle–brachial pressure index [ABPI])
- Respiratory conditions (e.g. pneumonia)
- Gastrointestinal (GI) conditions (e.g. obstruction, ileus)
- Neurological conditions (e.g. arteriovenous [AV] fistula)

Operative

- Confirm placement of the endotracheal tube

Post-operative

Assessment of organ systems:

- Cardiovascular conditions (i.e. pulmonary oedema)
- Blood pressure measurement
- Respiratory conditions (i.e. pneumonia, atelectasis)
- Gastrointestinal conditions (i.e. obstruction, ileus and nasogastric tube placement)

STOMAS

What is a stoma?

In medicine, a stoma (Greek – pl. stomata) is an opening, either natural or surgically created, which connects a portion of a cavity to another area.

A natural stoma is any opening in the body, such as the mouth. Any hollow organ can be manipulated into an artificial stoma. Surgical procedures that create stomas begin with a prefix denoting the organ, or area, being operated on and end with the suffix '-ostomy'.

What are the uses of a stoma?

- Feeding
- Lavage
- Exteriorisation
- Decompression, Diversion & Drainage

(*Please remember the mnemonic:* FLED)

What are the different types of stomas?

- Temporary or permanent
- End or loop
- Based on anatomical location

(i.e. tracheostomy, pharyngostomy, oesophagostomy, gastrostomy, duodenostomy, jejunostomy, ileostomy, colostomy, caecostomy, urostomy, nephrostomy)

How do you choose an abdominal stoma site?

Pre-operatively, the stoma site is marked on the skin whilst the patient is standing and sitting. The selected site should be away from the potential surgical incision, umbilicus and bony points. A stoma nurse should be involved in the patient's overall care (Figures 4.4 and 4.5).

Intra-operatively, a stoma should be created without tension, with viable bowel and with an adequate vascular supply.

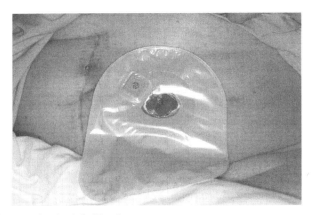

Figure 4.4 A colostomy in the left iliac fossa.

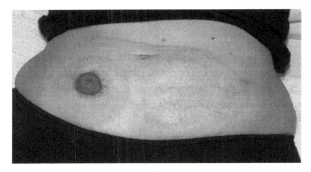

Figure 4.5 Spouted ileostomy in the right iliac fossa.

What are the potential complications of stomas?

- Immediate
  - Bleeding
  - Ischaemia
  - Necrosis
- Early
  - High output
  - Obstruction
  - Retraction
- Late
  - Obstruction
  - Prolapse
  - Retraction
  - Stenosis
  - Parastomal hernia
  - Skin excoriation and hypersensitivity
  - Electrolyte disturbance
  - Fistula formation
  - Stone (renal and gallstones) formation
  - Psychological and psychosexual complications

DRAINS

How are drains used in surgery?

Drainage can be established operatively be channelling the contents of the internal organs externally (i.e. ileostomy, colostomy, urostomy, cholecystectomy) or by diverting the visceral contents internally (i.e. gastric drainage via pyloroplasty or gastroenterostomy, cholecystojejunostomy or ureterosigmoidostomy).

Drains can be used to remove:

- Normal organ contents (i.e. Foley's catheter – Urine, nasogastric tube: gastric contents, extraventricular drains: cerebrospinal fluid (CSF) and chest drain: pleural fluid)
- Abnormal organ contents – (i.e. pus, blood and air)

What are the indications for inserting drains in surgery?

- Removal of harmful substances (i.e. nidus of infection)
- Removal of dead space (i.e. third space pooling)
- Monitor and prevent operative complications (i.e. haemorrhage and anastomotic leak)
- Creating a therapeutic tract (i.e. t-tube tract)

What are the different types of drains?

Active systems

- Open – Sump drain (an inner tube under suction is protected from blockage by an outer vented/irrigated tube)
- Closed – Redivac drain and chest drain (connected to an underwater seal)

Passive systems

- Open – Ribbon gauze wick, seton and corrugated drain
- Closed – Robinson drain

What are the potential complications of surgical drains?

- Infection
- Damage to surrounding structures – Bowel (anastomotic leakage, perforation, fistula formation), vessels (bleeding), nerves (motor and sensory disruption)
- Obstruction
- Migration
- Displacement

ADHESIONS

What are adhesions?

The union of two normally separate surfaces connected by fibrous connective tissue in an inflamed or damaged region. Adhesions may be classified into various types by virtue of whether they are early (fibrinous) or late (fibrous), or by underlying aetiology.

What do adhesions cause?

The most common adhesion-related problem is small-bowel obstruction (Figures 4.6 and 4.7). Adhesions are the commonest cause of intestinal obstruction in the developed world and are responsible for 60–70% of small-bowel obstruction. In addition, adhesions are implicated as a cause of chronic pain and abdominal pain and secondary infertility.

How do you classify adhesions?

- *Congenital (2%)*
  - Meckel's diverticulum
  - Malrotation of colon
  - Congenital bands

- *Acquired (98%)*
  - Post-operative (80%)
  - Post-inflammatory (18%)
  - Acute appendicitis, diverticulitis, cholecystitis, pelvic infection and inflammatory bowel disease (Crohn's disease and ulcerative colitis)

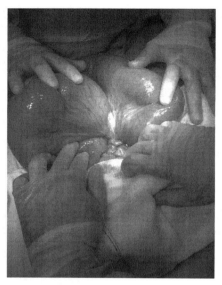

Figure 4.6 Band adhesion causing closed-loop obstruction.

How do you treat adhesions?

Pre-operative:

- Conservative treatment – Nasogastric suction and IV fluids ('drip and suck')
- Nutrition support

Operative:

- Surgical relief – Bypass, resection and adhesiolysis
- Preventative measures to avoid further adhesions (practical and theoretical):
  - Use of powder free gloves
  - Minimal handling of bowel
  - Instillation of various fluids (dextran 70, iodine) or gas into the peritoneal cavity to hold damaged surfaces apart
  - Enhancement of peristalsis to disrupt early fibrinous adhesions which have the potential to become fibrous adhesions if left
  - Covering anastomosis and raw peritoneal surfaces with inert membranes, lubricants or grafts of peritoneum (e.g. greater omentum placed between the bowel and abdominal wall)
  - Use of enzymes to digest adhesions (e.g. trypsin and hyaluronidase)
  - Instillation of substances to inhibit deposition of fibrin (fibrinolytic agents, steroids)

Post-operative:

- Conservative treatment – Nasogastric suction and IV fluids ('drip and suck')
- Nutrition support

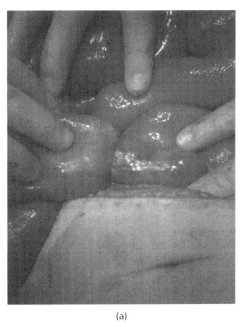

(a)

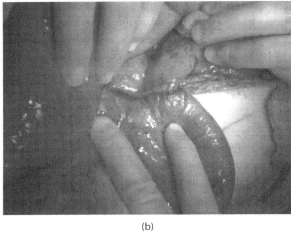

(b)

Figure 4.7 (a) and (b) Wall injury resulting from band compression, oversewn with an absorbable seromuscular suture.

- Antibiotics (if clinically indicated)
- Early mobilisation
- Early use of enteral feeding

SUDDEN DEATH IN SURGERY

What are the causes of sudden death in surgery?

Anaesthetic causes

Hypoxia:

- Respiratory obstruction (including kinked or displaced endotracheal tube)
- Vagal stimulation
- Disconnection from ventilator
- Tension pneumothorax secondary to positive pressure ventilation
- Mendelson syndrome or chemical pneumonitis (due to hydrochloric acid aspiration during anaesthetics)
- Shock (i.e. undetected hypotension secondary to internal bleeding)
- Embolisation (venous, air, fat)

Medication:

- Inappropriate drugs administered
- Anaphylactic reaction (i.e. drugs or blood)
- Overdose of medication (i.e. local anaesthetic)
- Cardiac dysrhythmias (vasodilators, ganglion blocks, diuretics)
- Electrolyte and metabolic imbalances
- Opiates

Surgical causes

- Hypotension (manipulation of bowel, mesenteric stretching or sympathectomy)
- Cardiac arrhythmias (induced by catheterisation, cardiac surgery)
- Oculocardiac reflex – (patient in prone position with direct pressure on eyes causing vagal stimulation)
- Damage to surrounding structures – Nerves, arteries and veins (e.g. incision of a groin aneurysm during a hernia repair)

Patient causes

- Myocardial infarction, pulmonary oedema, PE, stroke, dehydration and electrolyte imbalances

NUTRITION*

What is the normal daily resting energy expenditure of a 70-kg man?

He uses 1800 kcal.

---

* For further reading, see *Bailey and Love's Short Practice of Surgery* 27th edition, Chapter 19, 'Nutrition and fluid therapy'.

What are the protein/nitrogen requirements for a healthy and critically ill patient?

- Healthy patient requires 0.15 g/kg/day of nitrogen.
- Critically ill patient requires 0.2–0.3 g/kg/day of nitrogen.

What routes of nutrition are available and why are they chosen?

- *Enteral nutrition* is used in patients with a normally functioning GI tract. Feeding routes – oral, nasogastric, nasojejunal, nasoduodenal and tube enterostomy.
- *Parenteral nutrition* is the treatment of choice in patients with catabolic states and non-functioning GI tracts (Figures 4.8 and 4.9).

If enteral feeding is preferred, what are the indications for total parenteral nutrition?

- Patient who cannot ingest food
- Anorexia
  - Neurological disorders
  - Posterior fossa cranial surgery
  - Head injuries
  - Coma ($\Downarrow$GCS)
  - Trauma and tumours (involving the maxilla, head or neck)
- Patients with a malfunctioning GI tract
  - Short-bowel syndrome secondary to small bowel resection
  - Fistula (enteroenteric, enterocolic, enterovesical, enterocutaneous)
  - Obstruction (GI tumours, strictures, adhesions, pyloric obstruction)

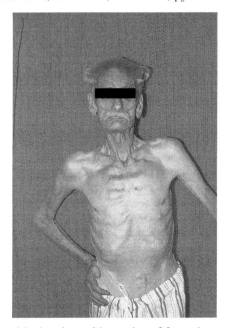

Figure 4.8 Severely malnourished patient with wasting of fat and muscle.

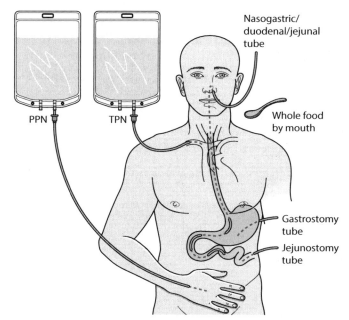

Figure 4.9 Techniques used for adjuvant nutritional support. PPN, partial parenteral nutrition; TPN, total parenteral nutrition. (Redrawn with permission from Rick Tharp, rxkinetics.com.)

- Paralytic ileus
- Inflammatory disease (Crohn's disease, ulcerative colitis, pancreatitis diverticular disease, radiation enteritis)
- Peptic ulceration
- Mesenteric vascular occlusion (ischaemia)
- Malignancy
- Trauma
- Hypercatabolic states
- Major GI anomalies (tracheo-oesphageal fistula, gastroschisis and intestinal atresia)

What are the major complications of enteral feeding?

Related to intubation of GI tract

- Fistulation
- Wound infection
- Peritonitis
- Displacement and catheter migration
- Obstruction of the tube

Related to delivery of nutrient to GI tract:

- Aspiration or pneumonia
- Feed intolerance
- Diarrhoea

What are the major complications of parenteral feeding?

Complications of parenteral nutrition

Related to nutrient deficiency

Related to catheter-mechanical:

- Blockage
- Migration
- Fracture
- Displacement
- Central vein thrombosis
- Air embolism
- Pneumothorax, haemothorax or hydrothorax
- Subclavian artery and vein injury
- Cardiac arrhythmias (if catheter is placed in the ventricle)

Related to catheter-infective:

- Exit site skin infection
- Line sepsis
- Infective endocarditis

Metabolic:

- Hyper- or hypo-glycaemia
- Hypertriglyceridaemia
- Hyperchloraemic acidosis
- Hypo-kalaemia, -magnesaemia and -phosphataemia
- Essential fatty acid deficiency
- Deranged liver function tests

METABOLIC RESPONSE TO SURGERY

What is the metabolic response to surgery?

The metabolic response to surgery is described by the 'ebb and flow' model (Figures 4.10 and 4.11).

Describe this model.

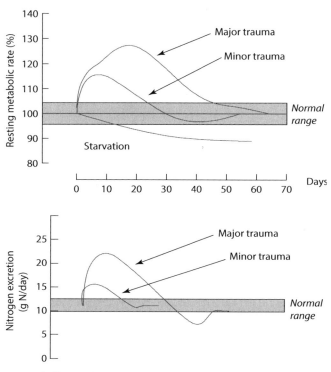

Figure 4.10 Hypermetabolism and increased nitrogen excretion are closely related to the magnitude of the initial injury and show a graded response.

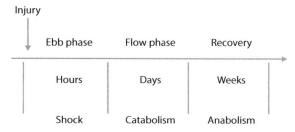

Figure 4.11 Phases of the physiological response to injury. (After Cuthbertson, DP, *Biochem J*, 24: 1244–1263, 1930.)

The Ebb phase

The 'Ebb phase' begins at the time of surgery (injury) and is characterised by hypovolaemia, depression of metabolic rate, reduced cardiac output, hypothermia, lactic acidosis and an overall reduction in energy expenditure. The main hormones in this phase are catecholamines, cortisol and aldosterone.

The Flow phase

This phase is divided into the catabolic and anabolic phases.

- In the *catabolic phase*, there is an increased catecholamine drive and energy is mobilised from adipose tissue and carbohydrate stores in the liver and muscle to aid recovery and repair. This phase is characterised by tissue oedema, increased metabolic rate, increased cardiac output, increased oxygen consumption and increased gluconeogenesis. Moreover, there is an increased production of hormones (catecholamines, cortisol, insulin, glucagons) and inflammatory cytokines (IL-1, IL-6, TNF-α) that utilises fat and protein stores. This leads to weight and nitrogen loss. The increased production of insulin results in insulin resistance. During this phase, the patient is at risk of infections and cardiac dysfunction.
- The *anabolic phase* occurs in conjunction with repair. There is weight gain, protein and fat stores increase, and the metabolic response returns to normal.

How long does each phase last?

The Ebb phase lasts 24–48 hours. The catabolic flow phase lasts between 3 and 10 days. The anabolic flow phase lasts from weeks to months.

What factors can be avoided to reduce the metabolic response to surgery?

- Continued haemorrhage (volume loss)
- Hypothermia
- Tissue oedema
- Poor tissue perfusion
- Starvation
- Immobility

How can surgical patients be optimised?

- Perform minimal access surgical techniques
- Block painful stimuli (adequate pain relief, including epidurals)
- Introduce beta-blockers and statins in appropriate patients (improve long-term outcomes)
- Avoid prolonged periods of stress and fasting
- Early mobilisation

SCREENING

What is screening?

Screening, in medicine, is a strategy used in a population to detect a disease in individuals without signs or symptoms of that disease. Unlike the rest of medicine, in screening, tests are performed on those patients without any clinical indication of disease.

What are the criteria needed for an effective screening programme?

1. The disease screened must be common and a significant problem in the population.
2. The natural history of the disease should be well understood with an early recognisable stage.
3. The test should be specific and sensitive.
4. The treatment should be effective.
5. The test must be acceptable.
6. There should be suitable facilities for the diagnosis and treatment.
7. There should be treatment available for the underlying condition.
8. The benefits of screening should outweigh the potential complications. Therefore, it should be safe.
9. The test should be cost effective.
10. Results should be audited according to the National Institute for Health and Clinical Excellence (NICE) guidelines.

What is sensitivity and specificity of a screening test?

Sensitivity is a measure of reliability of a screening test based on the proportion of people with a specific disease who react positively to the test (the higher the sensitivity the fewer false negatives). Sensitivity: True positives/Total number of final diagnosis positives.

Specificity is the proportion of people free from disease who react negatively to the test (the higher the specificity the fewer the false positives). Specificity: True negatives/Total number of final diagnosis negatives.

What examples of screening do you know?

- The Mantoux is a diagnostic tool to screen for exposure to tuberculosis.
- Alpha-fetoprotein screening is used to detect certain foetal abnormalities in pregnant women.
- Cancer screening is an attempt to prevent cancer, or diagnose it in its early stages. For example, the Pap smear is used to detect potentially precancerous lesions and prevent cervical cancer.

Name a current screening programme available in the England?

In 1988, the National Health Service (NHS) breast screening programme was introduced. It provides free breast screening (mammography) every 3 years for all women over 50 years of age. In addition, the NHS abdominal aortic aneurysm programme was established in 2009 and has been offered throughout the United Kingdom since the end of 2013. Men over 65 years of age are offered a screening abdominal ultrasound.

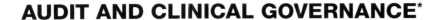

AUDIT AND CLINICAL GOVERNANCE*

What is an audit?

It is a systematic process by which a group of professionals review a current system of practice to identify weakness, make changes and monitor the standard of practice.

According to the National Institute for Clinical Excellence, it is 'a quality improvement process that seeks to improve patient care and outcome through systematic review of care against explicit criteria and the implementation of change'.

What types of audit do you know?

- *Standards-based audit* – A cycle which involves defining standards, collecting data to measure current practice against those standards and implementing any changes deemed necessary.
- *Peer review* – An assessment of the quality of care provided by a clinical team with a view to improving clinical care. Peers discuss individual cases.
- *Adverse occurrence screening and critical incident monitoring* – This is used to peer review cases, which had adverse or unexpected outcomes. A multidisciplinary team discusses individual cases, addresses the way the team functioned and what can be learnt for the future.
- *Patient surveys and focus groups* – Allows patients' views about the quality of care to be heard.

What is the audit cycle?

The clinical audit cycle is a systematic process of establishing best practice; measuring against criteria, taking action to improve care and monitoring to achieve improvement.

- Stage 1 – Identify the problem
- Stage 2 – Define criteria & standards
- Stage 3 – Data collection
- Stage 4 – Compare performance with criteria and standards
- Stage 5 – Implementing change
- Stage 6 – Re-audit: close the audit loop

What is clinical governance?

Clinical governance is the term used to describe a systematic approach of maintaining and improving the quality of patient care within a health-care system. According to Scally and Donaldson (1988), it is 'a framework through which NHS organisations are accountable for continually improving the quality of their services and safeguarding high standards of care by creating an environment in which excellence in clinical care will flourish'. There are three key attributes:

---

* For further reading, see *Bailey & Love's Short Practice of Surgery* 27th edition, Chapter 11, 'Surgical audit'.

- Maintaining high standards of care
- Transparent responsibility and accountability for standards
- Aim for constant improvement

What are the seven pillars of clinical governance?

- Audit
- Education and training – Continuing professional development
- Clinical effectiveness and research (evidence-based medicine)
- Risk management
- Patient and public involvement
- Information technology
- Staff management

RESEARCH AND STATISTICS*

What is a 'controlled clinical trial'?

A controlled trial is a scientific experiment in which one or more treatments are compared with a control treatment. The controls may be non-treatment, placebo or a standard clinical practice.

What is a crossover design for clinical trials?

In crossover designs, the patient acts as his or her own control. Treatments are compared and their order is randomised.

What is randomisation?

Randomisation is a method of assigning subjects to an experimental or control arm of a study. Each patient has an equal chance of appearing in either treatment group. It helps to avoid selection bias.

What is meant by blinding?

A method used to eliminate any bias inherent in the data collection. A study is single-blinded if the patient is unaware of the treatment allocation. In the best randomised controlled trials, neither patient nor researcher is aware of which therapy has been used until after the study has been conducted (double-blinded).

What are type I and type II errors?

- Type I errors occur when the null hypothesis (H_0) is rejected, when it is true. In otherwords, benefit is perceived when really there is none (false positive).
- Type II errors occur when the null hypothesis (H_0) is not rejected, when it is false. In other words, benefit is missed when it was there to be found (false negative).

---

* For further reading, see *Bailey & Love's Short Practice of Surgery* 27th edition, Chapter 11, 'Surgical audit'.

What is the power of a trial?

The power of the trial measures the sensitivity of the trial to detect a difference and is equal to 1-β, where β is the type II error rate.

What does it mean that a result is 'statistically significant'?

The result that is unlikely to have occurred by chance. Normally this equates to a *p* value of less than .05 (5%).

What is a 'confidence interval'?

Confidence interval (CI) is an interval estimate of a population parameter. It is used to indicate the reliability of an estimate. The CI provides the probability that a true population is contained within a range from a sample mean and its standard error.

Disease				
		+	**-**	
Test	+	True positives (a)	False positives (b)	PPV= a/a + b
	−	False negatives (c)	True negatives (d)	NPV=d/c + d
		Sensitivity= a/a + c	Specificity= d/d + b	

FRACTURES*

What is a fracture?

A fracture is a break in the continuity of the bone. It may be complete or incomplete (based on whether both cortices are involved), or open or closed (based on whether the overlying skin is intact). Descriptive terms for fractures are shown in Figure 4.12.

What are the phases of bone healing?

- *Reactive phase* – Fracture and inflammatory phase, followed by granulation tissue formation
- *Reparative phase* – Callus formation and lamellar bone deposition
- *Remodelling phase* – Remodelling to the original bone contour

What classification do you know for proximal femoral fractures?

The Garden Classification

        Stage I – Incomplete fractures (including impacted valgus fracture)
        Stage II – Complete fracture without displacement
        Stage III – Complete fracture with partial displacement
        Stage IV – Complete fracture with full displacement

---

* For further reading, see *Bailey & Love's Short Practice of Surgery* 27th edition, *Part* 5 'Elective Orthopaedics'

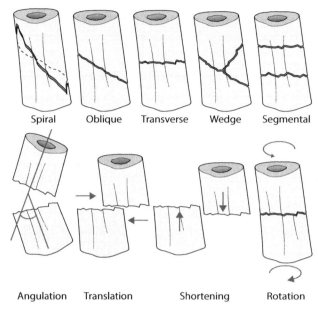

Spiral Oblique Transverse Wedge Segmental

Angulation Translation Shortening Rotation

Figure 4.12 Descriptive terms for fractures.

How may fractures be treated?

The treatment of bone fractures depends upon the type and location of the fracture and the patient's age and medical history. However, four phases can be identified (4 R's):

- *Resuscitation*
- *Reduction* (open or closed)
- *Restriction (immobilisation)* (cast splintage, functional bracing, continuous traction, internal fixation, external fixation)
- *Rehabilitation* (Physiotherapy)

What are the complications of fractures?

Early complications

Local:

- Vascular injury causing haemorrhage (internal or external)
- Visceral injury causing damage to the surrounding organs (i.e. brain, lung or bladder)
- Damage to surrounding soft tissue, nerves or skin
- Haemarthrosis
- Compartment syndrome (or Volkmann's ischaemia)
- Wound infection

Systemic:

- Fat embolism
- Shock
- Thromboembolism (pulmonary or venous)
- Exacerbation of underlying diseases (diabetes, ischaemic heart disease)
- Pneumonia

Late complications

Local:

- Delayed union
- Non-union
- Mal-union
- Joint stiffness
- Contractures
- Infection
- Myositis ossificans
- Avascular necrosis
- Algodystrophy (Sudeck's atrophy)
- Osteomyelitis
- Growth disturbance or deformity

Systemic:

- Gangrene, tetanus, septicaemia
- Fear of mobilising (compensation neurosis)
- Osteoarthritis

STERILISATION

What is meant by cleaning?

Cleaning is the process of physical removal of organic debris (e.g. blood, tissue and other body fluids) but does not necessarily destroy microorganisms.

What is disinfection?

Disinfection reduces the number of viable organisms.

What is sterilisation?

Sterilisation refers to the process that kills or eliminates transmissible viable microorganisms (i.e. bacteria, viruses, fungi, spores, cysts).

How may the methods of sterilisation be classified?

Physical sterilisation:

- Heat sterilisation
- Moist heat (pressurised steam autoclaves) 134°C
- Dry heat – 160°C
- Radiation sterilisation

Chemical sterilisation:

- Ethylene oxide˙
- Ozone
- Chlorine bleach
- Formaldehyde
- Glutaraldehyde
- Hydrogen peroxide
- Peracetic acid
- Ethanol (70%)

Give some examples of sterilisation?

- Moist heat sterilisation (steam autoclaves) – Trays of surgical instruments
- Dry heat sterilisation – Non-aqueous liquids and ointments
- Ionising radiation – Swabs, catheters, syringes
- Ethylene oxide – Sutures, electrical equipment
- Formaldehyde – Plastics
- Glutaraldehyde – Endoscopes

Does sterilisation destroy prions?

No

Prior to sterilisation of your surgical instruments, what do you need to do?

All instruments need to be cleaned and thoroughly dried before they are sterilised. There are three main cleaning methods: Hand scrubbing, ultrasonic cleaning and automated washing.

What types of disinfectants do you use when scrubbing? (Table 4.1)

- *2% chlorhexidine gluconate* is an aqueous quaternary ammonium compound. It has a residual effect and is effective for more than 4 hours. It has potent antiseptic activity against Gram-positive and Gram-negative organisms and some viruses, but only moderate activity against the tubercle bacillus. It has poor activity against spores and fungi.
- *7.5% povidone-iodine* is a potent bactericidal, fungicidal and virucidal agent. There is some activity against bacterial spores and good activity against tubercle bacilli. The iodine penetrates cell walls to produce anti-microbial effects. Iodine

Scrubbing up (Figure 4.13)

- Hat, mask and eye protection should be worn and jewellery should be removed prior to scrubbing.
- Nails and deep skin creases are cleaned for 1–2 minutes using a brush.
- Hands and forearms are washed systematically three times, the hands being held above the level of the elbows throughout.
- Hands and arms are dried from distal to proximal using a sterile towel.
- The folded gown is lifted away from the trolley and allowed to unfold (inside facing the wearer), whilst the top is held.
- Arms are inserted into the armholes simultaneously, hands remaining inside the gown until gloves are donned: The gown is secured by an unscrubbed staff member.
- Gloves are put on using a one- or two-person technique: From this point on, hands remain above waist level at all times.

Table 4.1 Classification of antiseptics commonly used in general surgical practice

Name	Presentation	Uses	Comments
Chlorhexidine (Hibiscrub)	Alcoholic 0.5% Aqueous 4%	Skin preparation Skin preparation. Surgical scrub in dilute solutions in open wounds	Has cumulative effect. Effective against Gram-positive organisms and relatively stable in the presence of pus and body fluids
Povidone-iodine (Betadine)	Alcoholic 10% Aqueous 7.5%	Skin preparation Skin preparation. Surgical scrub in dilute solutions in open wounds	Safe, fast-acting, broad spectrum. Some sporicidal activity. Anti-fungal iodine is not free but combined with polyvinylpyrrolidone (povidone)
Cetrimide (Savlon)	Aqueous	Handwashing Instrument and surface cleaning	*Pseudomonas* spp. may grow in stored contaminated solutions. Ammonium compounds have good detergent action (surface-active agent)
Alcohols	70% ethyl, isopropyl	Skin preparation	Should be reserved for use as disinfectants
Hypochlorites	Aqueous preparations (Eusol, Milton, Chloramine T)	Instrument and surface cleaning (debriding agent in open wounds)	Toxic to tissues
Hexachlo rophane	Aqueous bisphenol	Skin preparation Handwashing	Has action against Gram-negative organisms

has some residual effects but these are not sustained for more than 4 hours. In addition, it may cause irritation to the skin or allergic reactions.

• *Alcohols* are rapid acting anti-microbial agents with broad-spectrum activity. They are effective in destroying Gram-positive and Gram-negative bacteria, fungi, viruses and tubercle bacilli. However, they are not sporicidal.

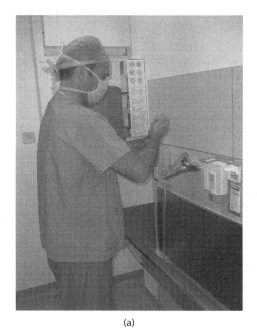

(a)

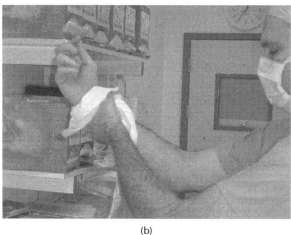

(b)

Figure 4.13 (a) and (b) Scrubbing up.

ANTIBACTERIAL PROPHYLAXIS

What is an antibiotic?

An antibiotic is a substance produced by or derived from a microorganism that destroys or inhibits the growth of other microorganisms.

How do you classify wound contamination?

Refer to Table 4.2.

What are the indications for antibacterial prophylaxis?

There is evidence to support the use of prophylactic antibiotics in clean-contaminated and contaminated operations. The indications for antibacterial prophylaxis can be classified as follows:

Endogenous contamination (after GI tract surgery) (Figure 4.14)

- Oesophageal and gastric surgery – Surgery for oesophagogastric carcinoma or gastric ulcers, patients on cimetidine, patients undergoing revision gastric surgery and in emergency conditions.

Table 4.2 Surgical site infection (SSI) rates relating to wound contamination

Type of surgery	Infection rate (%)	Rate before prophylaxis
Clean (no viscus opened)	1–2	Unchanged
Clean-contaminated (viscus-opened with minimal spillage)	<10	Gastric surgery up to 30%
		Biliary surgery up to 20%
Contaminated	15–20	Variable up to 60%
Dirty (pus, perforation or incision through an abscess)	<40	Up to 60% or more

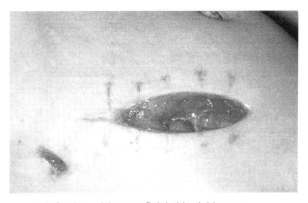

Figure 4.14 Major wound infection with superficial skin dehiscence.

- Biliary tract surgery – Risk factors include emergency surgery, > 70 years of age, jaundice, obesity, exploration of the common bile duct and concomitant alimentary procedures, biliary instrumentation without surgery (i.e. endoscopic retrograde cholangiopancreatography [ERCP]).
- Colorectal surgery – Surgery involving the bowel has a high rate of primary or secondary sepsis associated with anastomotic dehiscence.
- Appendicectomy
- Vaginal or abdominal hysterectomy
- Urogenital surgery

Exogenous contamination:

- Lower limb surgery in the presence of peripheral vascular disease
- Prosthetic joint replacements
- Prosthetic heart valves
- Neurosurgical shunts
- Extensive trauma and burns
- Surgical procedures and instrumentation in rheumatic and valvular heart disease
- Mesh insertion in hernia repair

Host immune system suppression:

- Diabetes mellitus
- Chronic renal failure
- Leukaemia
- Aplastic anaemia
- Malnourishment
- Carcinomatosis
- Obstructive jaundice
- Steroids therapy (Figure 4.15)
- Chemotherapy
- Cytotoxics

What is your choice of antibiotics for prophylaxis?

Choice of antibiotics for prophylaxis

- Empirical cover against expected pathogens with local hospital guidelines.
- Single-shot IV administration at induction of anaesthesia.
- Repeat only during long operations or if there is excessive blood loss.
- Continue as therapy if there is unexpected contamination or if a prosthetic is implanted in a patient with a septic source.
- Benzylpenicillin should be used if Clostridium gas gangrene infection is a possibility.
- Patients with heart valve disease or a prosthesis should be protected from bacteraemia caused by dental work, urethral instrumentation or visceral surgery.

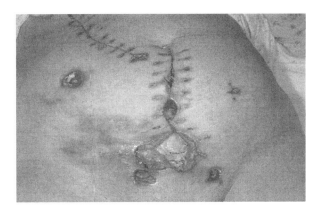

Figure 4.15 Delayed healing relating to infection in a patient on high-dose steroids.

DIABETES IN SURGERY

What are the complications that occur in patients with diabetes?

- Cardiovascular – Hypertension, angina and atherosclerosis
- Cerebrovascular – Stroke
- Peripheral vascular – Large blood vessel diseases (macroangiopathy), gangrene
- Renal – Uraemia and hypertension
- Eyes – Proliferative and non-proliferative retinopathies and cataracts
- Metabolic – Hyperglycaemia and ketoacidosis
- Nerves – Peripheral neuropathy (increased risk of pressure sores)
- Skin – Poor wound healing and infections

How should a diabetic patient be managed during surgery?

Pre-operative period:

- The aim is to prevent ketosis and avoid hypoglycaemia. Full medical assessment is performed to evaluate diabetic control and identify potential complications.
- Routine bloods should be sent (group and save [G&S], full blood count [FBC], urea and electrolyte [U&E], glucose, C-reactive protein [CRP], fasting glucose, glycated haemoglobin).
- A patient should not fast for prolonged periods, they should be scheduled first on an operating list.
- Diet-controlled diabetic patients
  - For minor surgery, no additional precautions are required.
  - For major surgery, monitor blood glucose and if elevated commence an insulin sliding scale.
- Oral hypoglycaemic-controlled diabetic patients

- For minor surgery, the morning dose of the oral hypoglycaemic agent should be omitted. It is restarted once the patient is eating and drinking. Continue to monitor blood glucose levels.
- For major surgery, patient should be commenced on an insulin sliding scale when they are nil by mouth and stopped when they have resumed eating and drinking.
- Insulin-controlled diabetic patients
  - For all surgeries, the insulin dose should not be given whilst the patient is fasted. They should be commenced on an insulin sliding scale with dextrose infusion. They may be stopped when the patient has resumed eating and drinking.

Intra-operative period:

- Anaesthesia combined with surgical stress has a definite hyperglycaemic effect.
- Consider local, regional, spinal or epidural anaesthesia. Moreover, a general anaesthetic is tolerated in most diabetics.
- BP and blood glucose should be monitored throughout surgery.

Post-operative period:

- Aim to have the patient's blood glucose levels within normal range.
- Oral fluids once started should be followed by a soft diet and then a diabetic diet.
- Normal regimes may then be resumed.
- Monitor for symptoms and signs of infection (Figure 4.16).

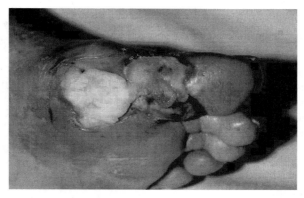

Figure 4.16 A severe diabetic foot infection, with marked infection, necrosis and soft–tissue loss. The patient was neuropathic but not ischaemic and it was possible to salvage a functional foot by 'filleting' the hallux and using the soft tissues to cover the defect.

HUMAN IMMUNODEFICIENCY VIRUS IN SURGERY

What is human immunodeficiency virus?

Human immunodeficiency virus (HIV) is a lentivirus (a member of the retrovirus family) that may lead to acquired immunodeficiency syndrome (AIDS). In 1981, AIDS was first identified in Los Angeles; the virus destroys helper (CD4) T-cells resulting in the suppression of the body's immune response.

Who is at high risk of acquiring the infection?

- Sexual activity – Unprotected sexual relations, including homosexual males
- Blood products – IV drug users, haemophiliacs (before 1985) and recipients of blood and blood products
- Mother-to-child – In utero, intrapartum and breast-feeding
- Endemic areas – Africa and Southeast Asia

How long does it take to 'seroconvert'?

In 85% of cases, seroconversion occurs within 12 weeks of infection.

How are doctors and other health workers at risk?

Whilst treating patients, we are commonly exposed to bodily fluids (including blood). This can occur with needle stick injuries, mucosal contact and bodily fluid spillages and splashes.

What is the risk of HIV transmission following exposure with infected blood?

Route	Estimated infections/10,000 exposures to an infected source	%
Blood transfusion	9000	90
Needle-sharing	67	0.67
Percutaneous needle stick	30	0.3

What factors increase the risk of sero-conversion following needle stick injuries?

- Exposure to large inoculation of blood
- Deep penetrating injury
- Visible blood on the needle
- Procedures that cannulate blood vessels (arterial blood gases [ABGs], central lines)
- Patient with high viral loads and low CD4 counts
- HIV progression (AIDS)

What universal precautions should be taken when operating on HIV positive patients?

- When there is a risk of splashing, particularly with power tools, use of a full face mask is recommended, or protective glasses.
- Use of fully waterproof, disposable gowns and drapes, particularly during seroconversion.
- Boots to be worn, not clogs, to avoid injury from dropping sharps.
- Double gloving (a larger size on the inside is more comfortable).
- Allow only essential personnel in theatre.
- Avoid unnecessary movement in theatre.
- Respect is required for sharps, with passage in a kidney dish.
- A slow meticulous operative technique is needed to minimise bleeding.

When do you consider administering post-exposure prophylaxis?

The uptake and processing of the HIV antigen may take several hours to days. There is a window of opportunity for prevention. In the United Kingdom, prophylaxis is recommended for high-risk individuals. A set protocol should be followed:

Immediate action

Following any exposure, the site is washed liberally with soap and water (without scrubbing). Free bleeding of puncture wounds should be encouraged. Exposed mucous membranes, including conjunctivae, should be irrigated copiously with water, before and after removing any contact lenses.

Risk assessment

This assessment needs to be made urgently by someone other than the exposed worker about the appropriateness of starting treatment. Consideration should also be given to risk of exposure to hepatitis B and C (the rule of 3's applies; for hepatitis B the risk of transmission following needle stick exposure from an infected source is approximately 30%, for hepatitis C the risk is approximately 3% and for HIV the risk is approximately 0.3%). The decision for prophylaxis is based on the exposure potential, the type of body fluid or substance involved, and the route and severity of the exposure. There are three types of exposure in health-care settings associated with significant risk:

- Percutaneous injury (from needles, instruments, bone fragments, significant bites which break the skin)
- Exposure of broken skin (abrasions, cuts, eczema)
- Exposure of mucous membranes (including the eye)

Prescribing PEP

Post-exposure prophylaxis (PEP) should be recommended to health-care workers if they have had a significant occupational exposure to blood, or high-risk body fluid from a patient, or other source, either known to be HIV infected, or considered to be at high risk of HIV infection. PEP is generally not offered after exposure through any route with low-risk materials (i.e. urine, vomit, saliva, faeces) unless they are visibly blood stained. It is important to take into account the views of the exposed health-care worker.

What is the recommended medication for PEP?

The recommended medication in PEP starter packs includes:

- Zidovudine 250 or 300 mg (b.d.)
- Lamivudine 150 mg (b.d.)
- Nelfinavir 1250 mg (b.d.) or 750 mg (t.d.s.)

VENOUS THROMBOEMBOLISM

What are the risk factors for venous thromboembolism?

The risk factors for venous thromboembolism (Figures 4.17 an 4.18) can be classified as follows:

- Primary (congenital) versus secondary (acquired)
- Patient-related versus surgical-related factors
- By Virchow's triad (problems with the vessel wall, the flow and the constituents of blood)
- Pre-operative versus intra-operative versus post-operative risk factors

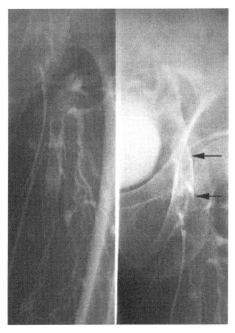

Figure 4.17 An ascending venogram of a deep vein thrombosis seen as filling defects (arrows) with contrast passing around the thrombus.

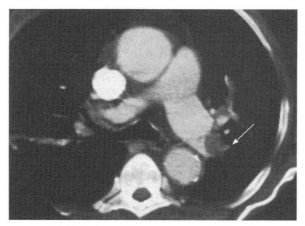

Figure 4.18 A computed tomography scan showing pulmonary emboli as filling defects (arrow) in the pulmonary artery.

Patient-related factors:

- Increasing age
- Previous or family history of DVT or PE
- Varicose veins
- Malignancy
- Obesity
- Immobility (including a lower limb plaster cast)
- Pregnancy
- Thrombophilia (e.g. factor V Leiden, Protein C/Protein S deficiency, lupus anticoagulant, antithrombin III deficiency, antiphospholipid antibody)
- High-dose oestrogen therapy (e.g. oral contraceptive pill)
- Smoking

Factors involving the disease or surgery:

- Trauma or surgery (especially abdominal, pelvic, hip or lower limb)
- Length of operation
- Malignancy
- Recent myocardial infarction
- Paralysis of lower limb
- Congestive heart failure
- Polycythaemia
- Paraproteinaemia
- Homocystinaemia
- Inflammatory bowel disease
- Nephrotic syndrome

How can venous thromboembolism be prevented around the time of surgery?

The answer can be classified as follows:

- Mechanical versus pharmacological prophylaxis
- Pre-operative versus intra-operative versus post-operative preventative strategies

Pre-operatively:

- Graduated elastic compression stockings (thromboembolic deterrent [TED] stocking)
- Intermittent pneumatic compression devices
- Low-molecular weight (LMW) heparin
- Fluids
- Stop smoking
- Stop oral contraceptive pill and hormone replacement therapy (HRT) 6 weeks prior to surgery
- Early mobilisation

Intra-operatively:

- Care in positioning, avoid pressure areas
- Gel pads
- TED stockings
- Pneumatic calf compression (Flowtron boots)
- Keep the patient well hydrated
- Keep time on the table to a minimum
- Neuraxial anaesthesia

Post-operatively:

- Early mobilisation with physiotherapy
- Elevating the feet and asking the patient not to cross their legs
- Low-molecular-weight heparin

Table 4.3 Modified Wells criteria for predicting pulmonary embolism

Variable	Points
Clinical signs and symptoms of DVT (minimum of leg swelling and pain on palpation of deep veins)	3.0
Alternative diagnosis less likely than PE	3.0
Heart rate >100	1.5
Immobilisation >3 days of surgery within past 4 weeks	1.5
Previous DVT or PE	1.5
Haemoptysis	1.0
Malignancy (treatment or palliation within past 6 months)	1.0

Abbreviations: DVT, deep venous thrombosis; PE, pulmonary embolism.

Note: A score of <4 means PE is unlikely, >4 is suggestive of PE.

- Dose-adjusted warfarin
- TED stockings
- Adequate hydration

What is the Modified Wells criteria for predicting PE?

Discuss the mechanism of action of the following: Heparin, LMW heparin and Warfarin.

Heparin

Increases affinity of antithrombin for thrombin and factor Xa

Leads to prolongation of the activated partial thromboplastin time (aPTT)

LMW heparin

Increases cleavage of factor Xa by antithrombin

No prolongation of the aPTT

Warfarin

Inhibits vitamin K-dependent epoxide reductase

Prevents conversion of vitamin K-dependent factors (factors II, VII, IX and X)

MONITORING DURING ANAESTHESIA

What types of monitoring do you know of?

- Invasive versus non-invasive
- Continuous versus intermittent

Examples:

- Intermittent, non-invasive – BP recordings with a sphygmomanometer, 12-lead electrocardiogram (ECG)
- Continuous, non-invasive – Pulse oximetry, cardiac monitor
- Intermittent, invasive – ABGs, blood glucose monitoring, hourly urine outputs
- Continuous, invasive – Invasive BP monitoring with an arterial line, end tidal CO_2, central venous lines, Swan-Ganz catheters

How do pulse oximeters work?

There are two principles involved:

- Differential light absorption by deoxyHb and oxyHb at two wavelengths, usually 660 nm (red, where deoxyHb > oxyHb) and 940 nm (near infrared, where oxyHb > deoxyHb).

- Identification of the pulsatile component of the signal. Since the pulsating blood in the artery is the only substance that is changing, the stable substances (skin, tissue etc.) are eliminated from the calculation.

What are the limitations and sources of error of pulse oximeters?

Limitations:

- Pulse oximetry tells you nothing about ventilation (CO_2).
- The oximeter progressively under-reads the saturation as the haemoglobin falls.
- There is a response delay (15–20 seconds).

Sources of error:

- Poor perfusion (constrictive clothing, BP cuffs) and hypothermia
- Artefact caused by motion, shivering and tremors
- Excessive ambient light causes spurious readings
- Venous pulsation (venous saturations are 75% so the effect is significant)
- Dyshaemoglobinaemias – Oxygen saturations are overestimated with carboxyHb (smokers, burns; oximeter detects COHb as oxyHb), underestimated with metHb (prilocaine; oxygen saturations tend towards 85%) and sulphaemoglobinaemia
- Vital dyes, nail varnish and skin pigmentation (deep jaundice underestimates the oxygen saturations)

What factors predispose the surgical patient to hypothermia?

- Long pre-operative fasting phase
- Anaesthesia induces loss of thermoregulatory control
- The effect of anaesthetic agents (peripheral vasodilatation)
- Exposure of skin and organs to a cold operating theatre
- Volatile skin preparation (which cools by evaporation)
- Infusion of cold IV fluids
- Prolonged immobility on the operating table
- Emergency surgery on shocked patients who are already hypothermic
- In children, the large surface area to weight ratio means that they can lose heat quickly

What are the consequences of peri-operative hypothermia?

- Increased surgical bleeding (the enzymes in the clotting cascade are slowed down)
- Increased incidence of myocardial infarcts and arrhythmias (hypothermia and shivering increases oxygen consumption and vascular resistance)
- Delayed recovery from anaesthetic/prolonged drug metabolism
- Excessive sympathetic nerve stimulation on waking
- Negative nitrogen balance (protein catabolism)

- Impaired immune function
- Increased wound infection
- Patient discomfort

Describe measures to reduce heat loss in patients undergoing surgery.

Environment:

- Increase ambient pressure and humidity

Patient:

- Cover patient during transfers and induction
- Warm all irrigation, IV fluids and blood
- Insulate patient with wrap/warming blanket
- Enclose exposed viscera in plastic bags
- Warm and humidify inspired gases
- Intra-operative use of forced air warming devices (Bair Huggers) (Figure 4.19)

POST-OPERATIVE COMPLICATIONS

You are working on the General Surgery Unit. The nurse bleeps you because she is worried about Mr. Jones, a 68-year-old gentleman, who underwent an anterior

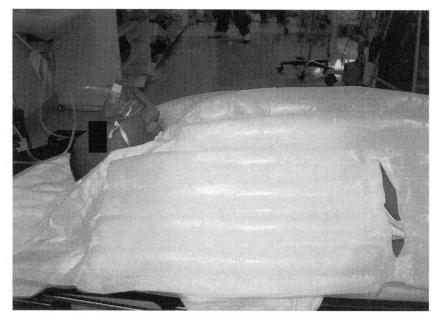

Figure 4.19 External warming blanket. (Courtesy of Johannesburg Hospital Trauma Unit.)

resection 7 days ago. You go to the ward to assess the patient and his wound (Figure 4.20).

Comment on your findings.

The observations chart shows a tachycardia, coupled with a low BP. The patient also has a low-grade fever.

What is the diagnosis?

Shock

What is shock?

Shock is the inadequate perfusion of tissues resulting in tissue hypoxia.

What types of shock do you know of?

- Hypovolaemic
- Septic
- Cardiogenic, i.e. pump failure (e.g. following a myocardial infarct)
- Obstructive, e.g. PE, cardiac tamponade, tension pneumothorax
- Neurogenic
- Anaphylactic
- Endocrine, e.g. Addisonian crisis

Why do you think this patient has most likely deteriorated?

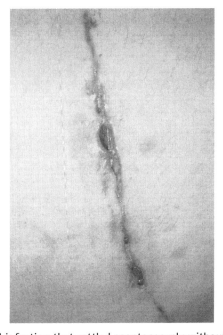

Figure 4.20 Minor wound infection that settled spontaneously without antibiotics.

Review the observations chart.

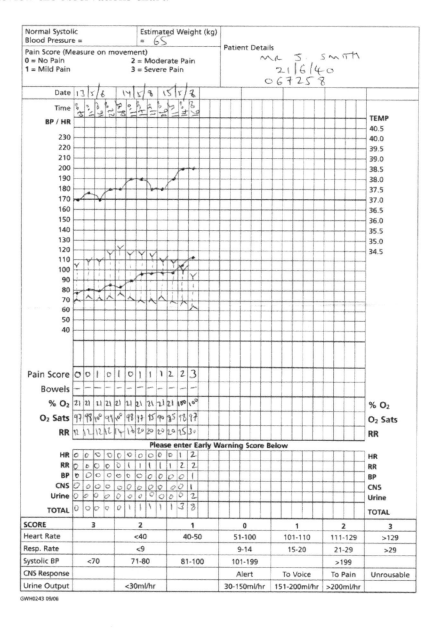

The most likely reasons are sepsis (including the presence of an intra-abdominal collection), a pulmonary embolus or an anastomotic leak. Bleeding is unlikely at day 7 post-operative and also note the patient has an associated fever. This patient is acutely unwell and requires urgent resuscitation and investigation to determine the cause (Table 4.4).

Table 4.4 Clinical features of shock

	Compensated	Mild	Moderate	Severe
Lactic acidosis	+	++	++	+++
Urine output	Normal	Normal	Reduced	Anuric
Conscious level	Normal	Mild anxiety	Drowsy	Comatose
Respiratory rate	Normal	Increased	Increased	Laboured
Pulse rate	Mild increase	Increased	Increased	Increased
Blood pressure	Normal	Normal	Mild hypotension	Severe hypotension

BLOOD TRANSFUSIONS

What are the complications of blood transfusions?

Acute complications

Immunological:

- Acute haemolytic transfusion reactions (ABO incompatibility)
- Febrile, non-haemolytic transfusion reactions
- Urticarial reactions
- Anaphylactic reactions
- Transfusion-related acute lung injury (TRALI)

Non-immunological:

- Bacterial contamination (sepsis)
- Congestive cardiac failure (CCF) (volume overload)
- Hypothermia
- Electrolyte disturbances ($\uparrow$K, $\downarrow$Ca, pH imbalances)
- Air embolism
- Coagulopathy

Delayed complications

Immunological:

- Delayed haemolytic transfusion reactions
- Graft versus host disease
- Iron overload
- Post-transfusion purpura
- Immune modulation

Non-immunological:

- Infections (Hepatitis B/C, HIV, human T-cell lymphotrophic virus [HTLV], cytomegalovirus [CMV], malaria, prions)

What are red blood cell antigens?

Human red blood cells have on their cell surface many different antigens. Two groups of red blood cell antigens are of major importance in the surgical setting-ABO and rhesus system (Figure 4.21).

ABO system

These are strongly antigenic and are associated with naturally occurring antibodies in the serum. The system is composed of three allelic genes-A, B and O, which control synthesis of enzymes that add carbohydrate residues to the cell surface glycoprotein. The system allows for six potential genotypes although there are only four possible phenotypes. Blood group O is the universal donor type, as it contains no antigens to provoke a reaction. Group AB individuals are universal recipients, as they have no circulating antibodies (Table 4.5).

Rhesus system

The rhesus D (Rh (D)) antigen is strongly antigenic and is present in approximately 85% of the population in the United Kingdom. Antibodies to the D antigen are

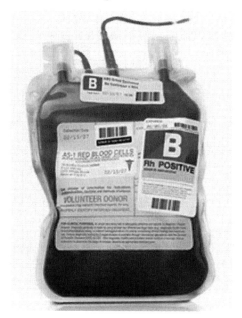

Figure 4.21 A blood transfusion bag.

Table 4.5 ABO blood group system

Phenotype	Genotype	Antigens	Antibodies	Frequency (%)
O	OO	O	Anti-A, anti-B	46
A	AA or AO	A	Anti-B	42
B	BB or BO	B	Anti-A	9
AB	AB	AB	None	3

not naturally present in the serum of the remaining 15% of individuals, but their formation may be stimulated by the transfusion of Rh-positive red cells, or acquired during the delivery of an Rh (D)-positive baby. Acquired antibodies can cross the placenta in pregnancy and if present in an Rh (D)-negative mother may result in severe haemolytic anaemia and even death (hydrops fetalis) in an Rh (D)-positive fetus *in utero*.

What is SHOT?

SHOT stands for 'serious hazards of transfusion', a national reporting body that collates anonymised data nationwide on serious adverse events of blood transfusions. An annual report is published and guidelines are issued to try and improve transfusion practice in hospitals nationwide.

What is the legal position on Jehovah's Witness patients and the use of blood products?

This is a difficult area. Wherever possible, consultants should be involved and a second medical opinion should be sought. In addition, the trust legal services department should be informed. The Royal College of Surgeons and the Association of Anaesthetists have produced guidelines:

Adults

- Competent adult patients of sound mind have the right to refuse medical treatment (however irrational this may be perceived to be) even if the consequences of such refusal may lead to the patient's death or serious injury.
- To administer blood in the face of refusal by a patient may be unlawful and could lead to criminal and/or civil proceedings.
- In an emergency if the patient is able to give an informed, rational opinion, or if an applicable advance directive exists, this should be acted upon.
- If this is not the case, the clinical judgement of a doctor should take precedence over the opinion of relatives or associates.

Children

In the case of children, the situation is more complicated:

- If a child needs blood in a life-threatening emergency, despite the surgeon's best efforts to contain haemorrhage, it should be given. The surgeon who stands by and allows a 'minor' patient to die in circumstances where blood might have avoided death may be vulnerable to criminal prosecution.
- Although children of 16 and over may consent to treatment, as can mature children under 16 (Gillick competency), this does not give such children the right to refuse treatment which is required in their best interests. However, it is always necessary to ascertain the views of the child so that they may be taken into account.
- In an elective, or semi-elective situation, where the child requires a blood transfusion, refusal by the parents may be overridden by an application to the High Court for an Order that the child receive a blood transfusion or other necessary medical treatment.

What strategies do you know of for avoiding or reducing the need for blood transfusions?

Blood substitution:

- Crystalloids and/or colloids
- Artificial blood substitutes (currently confined to clinical trials)

Pharmacological methods:

- Ferrous sulphate
- Antifibrinolytics such as tranexamic acid or desmopressin
- Erythropoietin
- Recombinant factor VIIa

Anaesthetic techniques:

- Anaesthetic techniques to reduce bleeding such as inducing hypotension or hypothermia

Surgical technique:

- Meticulous haemostasis at surgery including the use of local haemostatics such as surgicel, fibrin glue and sealants

Autologous transfusion:

- Pre-operative autologous blood donation
- Acute normovolaemic haemodilution
- Intra-operative and post-operative cell salvage techniques

DAY CASE SURGERY

What are the advantages and disadvantages of day case surgery?

Advantages:

- Release of inpatient beds (resources)
- Increase the potential number of patients treated
- Greater efficiency of operating list scheduling
- A firm date and time for operation with reduced cancellation risk
- Reduced disruption to patient's lives
- Reduced incidence of nosocomial infections
- Cost efficacy

Disadvantages:

- Requirement for adequate aftercare
- Experienced and trained surgical and anaesthetic staff mandatory
- Requirement for inpatient admission or readmission in cases of unexpected complications, inadequate analgesia etc.

What are the criteria for day case surgery?

Patient-related factors:

- American Society of Anaesthesiologists (ASA) class I or II
- Body mass index (BMI) < 35
- Patient acceptability
- Psychologically suitable patient

Surgical factors:

- Operation < 1 hour duration
- An operation that is not associated with:
  - Significant blood loss or fluid shifts
  - Significant nausea and vomiting
  - Pain that cannot be treated with simple analgesia
  - Prolonged immobilisation
- An operation that has a low morbidity with a low incidence of post-operative complications

Social factors:

- The patient lives < 1 hour drive from the unit
- Someone to drive the patient home after surgery

- A responsible adult to supervise the patient at home for the first 24–48 hours post-operatively
- The patient has access to a telephone, lift (for an upper floor flat) and toilet at home

What is the American Society of Anaesthesiologists (ASA) Physical Status Classification?

1. A normal health patient

2. A patient with mild systematic disease

3. A patient with severe systemic disease

4. A patient with severe systemic disease that is a constant threat to life

5. A moribund patient who is not expected to survive without the operation

THE MULTIPLY INJURED PATIENT: ADVANCED TRAUMA LIFE SUPPORT – PRINCIPLES AND PRACTICE*

Bear in mind that you may be faced with a resuscitation, or Advanced Trauma Life Support (ATLS), scenario as in the trauma 'moulage' scenarios of the ATLS course and it will be well worth your time recapping on the principles of ATLS prior to your exam, which we have done for you here.

How would you manage a multiply injured patient who was brought in to the emergency department following a road traffic accident?

The patient would need to be assessed according to the principles of ATLS. This would involve the following (Figures 4.22 and 4.23):

Primary survey:

- Airway with cervical spine protection
- Breathing and ventilation
- Circulation and haemorrhage control
- Disability (neurological status)
- Exposure and environment

Adjuncts to primary survey:

- Monitoring tools – Pulse oximetry, BP, CO_2 monitor, ECG, cardiac monitor, ABG, temperature probe

---

* For further reading, see *Bailey and Love's Short Practice of Surgery* 27th edition, Chapter 22, 'Introduction to trauma' and Chapter 23, 'Early assessment and management of trauma'.

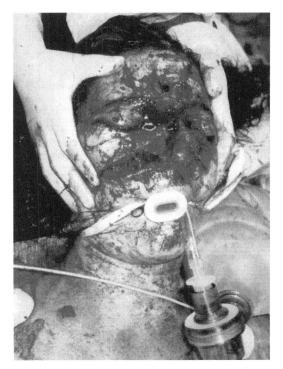

Figure 4.22 Unrestrained driver with severe craniofacial injury. (Courtesy of Johannesburg Hospital Trauma Unit.)

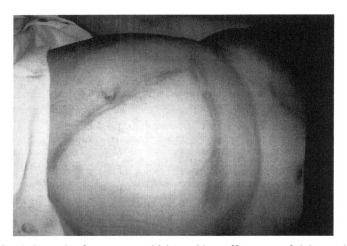

Figure 4.23 Seatbelt mark after motor vehicle accident. (Courtesy of Johannesburg Hospital Trauma Unit.)

- Blood tests – Glucose (finger-prick test), FBC, U&Es, amylase, clotting screen, toxicology, cross-match, including a pregnancy test for all females of child-bearing age
- Two wide-bore cannulae for IV fluids
- Analgesia (often neglected)
- Urinary catheter, if not contraindicated
- Nasogastric tube, if not contraindicated
- X-rays (trauma series) – Lateral C-spine (including T1 vertebra), anterior and posterior (AP) chest and AP pelvis
- Other radiological investigations – Abdominal ultrasound scan (Focussed Assessment with Sonography for Trauma [FAST] scan), diagnostic peritoneal lavage, computed tomography (CT) scan (if patient stable)
- Reassess primary survey and consider need for transfer

AMPLE history:

- Allergies
- Medications
- Past medical and surgical history/Pregnancy
- Last meal and fluid/Last tetanus
- Events/Environment related to the injury

Secondary survey:
- A full head-to-toe evaluation of the patient to ensure no injury is missed.
- Log-roll – Examine the back and perform a rectal examination at the same time.

Further evaluation:

- Carry out continuous assessment and reassessment of the patient to detect any changes in their condition
- Documentation and legal considerations
- Definitive care and transfer

CHAPTER 5: CRITICAL CARE

THE CRITICAL CARE OSCE

Critical care is examined by direct viva and through written questions. An understanding of basic physiological principles is essential to competently answer the probing management-style questions.

AIRWAYS AND VENTILATION

How would you assess a patient's airway?
  • 'Look' – Symmetrical chest wall movement, use of accessory muscles, foreign body in the airway, 'see-saw' breathing
  • 'Listen' – Coughing, gagging, choking, stridor, gurgling
  • 'Feel' – Chest wall movements, oronasal air flow
What options do you have to manage the airway?
  • Manoeuvres – Suction, head-tilt, chin lift, jaw thrust
  • Adjuncts – Oro/naso-pharyngeal airways
  • Definitive – Oro/naso-tracheal intubation, surgical airway (cricothyroidotomy, tracheostomy)
What types of tracheostomy do you know of?
  • Elective versus emergency
  • Cuffed versus uncuffed
  • Fenestrated versus unfenestrated
  • Open versus percutaneous
  • Silver metal versus plastic
What complications should you be aware of with a tracheostomy?
  • Bleeding – May aspirate
  • Subcutaneous emphysema
  • Local infection
  • Tracheal stenosis
  • Damage to brachiocephalic vein from misplacement with tube change
How might you assist ventilation?
  • Non-invasive positive pressure ventilation, e.g. bi-level positive airway pressure (BIPAP), continuous positive airway pressure (CPAP)
  • Invasive positive pressure ventilation
Which patients may benefit from non-invasive positive pressure ventilation?
  • Exacerbation of chronic obstructive pulmonary disease (COPD)
  • Acute pulmonary oedema
  • Pneumonia
  • Facilitation of weaning from mechanical (invasive) ventilation
What types of mechanical ventilators do you know and how do they work?
  • Types – Volume-cycled (delivers preset volume), pressure-cycled (delivers preset pressure), flow-cycled (delivers preset flow) and time-cycled (delivers preset frequency)

- Modes – Controlled mechanical or continuous mandatory (ventilates regardless of inspiratory effort), assist-controlled (ventilates in response to inspiratory effort and if absent effort), synchronous intermittent (ventilates supplementary to spontaneous breathing)
- Adjuncts – Positive end-expiratory pressure (PEEP), CPAP

ACID–BASE

Can you interpret this arterial blood–gas profile? (Figure 5.1)

What could be causing it?

- Respiratory acidosis – Hypoventilation which has both central (depression of the respiratory centres, e.g. opioids, GAs) and peripheral causes (acute respiratory failure (type II), airway obstruction and decreased chest wall movement, e.g. trauma)
- Metabolic acidosis can be classified into

Raised anion gap?

- Raised lactic acid (secondary to shock, infection and hypoxia)
- Raised ketoacids (secondary to diabetes mellitus, alcohol)
- 'Fixed' acids (renal failure)
- Ingested acids (drugs and toxins)

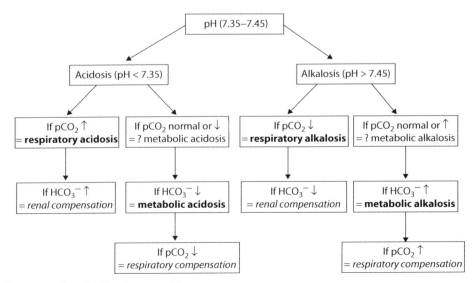

Figure 5.1 Arterial blood–gas profile.

Normal anion gap (e.g. diarrhoea, fistulae, renal tubular acidosis etc?)

- Respiratory alkalosis – Hyperventilation (e.g. fever, sepsis, pain, anxiety, pneumonia, pulmonary embolus etc.)
- Metabolic alkalosis – Excess loss of acid (e.g. vomiting)

What are the commonest causes of new onset dyspnoea several days post-op? How would you investigate and treat it?

- Pulmonary embolism (PE), pneumonia, myocardial infarction (MI) and pulmonary oedema, bronchospasm, pneumothorax
- History and physical examination
- Arterial blood gas (ABG)
- Blood profile – Haematology (raised white cell count [WCC]), C-reactive protein (CRP), coagulation (D-dimer)
- Chest x-ray (CXR)
- Electrocardiogram (ECG)
- V/Q, computed tomography pulmonary angiogram (CTPA)
- Deep vein Doppler
- Pneumonia – Antibiotics
- PE – Anticoagulation

You are having a busy weekend on call and your FY1 has just returned from seeing a patient with a history of alcoholic liver disease and atrial fibrillation, now presenting with non-specific abdominal pain. Your FY1 hands you the patient's arterial blood–gas profile whilst telling you the patient is a poor historian and is being disruptive in A&E. What do you make of these ABGs?

pH	7.32
PCO_2	3.43 kPa
PO_2	14.4 kPa
HCO_3^-	17 mmol/L

This is a metabolic acidosis with respiratory compensation.

Your FY1 has almost lost his patience with this patient and feels that the patient is just intoxicated. Do you agree? What would you do next?

- The patient may well be intoxicated but he has a metabolic acidosis. In view of the clinical history and symptoms and signs, bowel ischaemia secondary to a mesenteric embolic event must be excluded.
- This is potentially a surgical emergency and thus the patient urgently needs resuscitating, a more senior surgical review, followed by CT imaging and laparotomy.

What else could you calculate? What else would you ask for?

- You could calculate the anion gap which you would expect to be raised.
- A lactate level would also be helpful.

BURNS

How would you assess a patient presenting with a burn injury?

- A, B, C
- Careful assessment for inhalational injury (facial burns, singed hair, cough, hoarseness, stridor, carbonaceous sputum) with a low threshold for intubation
- Wallace's rule of nines (head 9%, single arm 9%, anterior trunk 18%, posterior trunk 18%, single leg 18%, genitalia 1%)
- Partial thickness (red/white, blistering, sensate) versus full thickness (white, leathery, desensate)
- Early discussion with burns unit to arrange transfer if necessary

How would you resuscitate them?

- In addition to maintenance fluid, replacement crystalloids are given at 4 mL/kg body weight/% burn of total body surface area over 24 hours (Parkland formula).
- 50% of the total calculated volume is given in the first 8 hours.

What complications should you be vigilant of?

- Shock from fluid and electrolyte losses
- Sepsis
- Acute respiratory distress syndrome (ARDS)
- Constricting effect of circumferential burns may cause ischaemia (e.g. if on the limbs) or ventilatory problems (e.g. if chest wall burns) which may require escharotomy (see Figure 5.2)
- Renal failure secondary to myoglobinuria

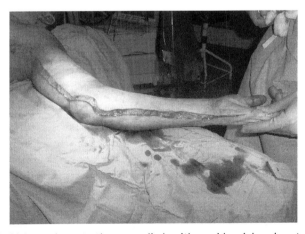

Figure 5.2 A full-thickness burn to the upper limb with a mid-axial escharotomy. The soot and debris have been washed off.

INTENSIVE CARE UNIT

Which patients are appropriate to be referred to the intensive care unit (ICU)?

- Those that need advanced respiratory support.
- Those that need mechanical support of two or more organ systems.
- Those that need close and/or invasive monitoring of organ dysfunction.
- Those that need intensive nursing input (usually one to one).
- Those where the condition is potentially *reversible.*

What is shock? What types do you know? How do you grade it?

- Inadequate tissue perfusion secondary to acute circulatory failure
- Hypovolaemic, septic, anaphylactic, cardiogenic, neurogenic
- Four grades of severity
  - Grade 1 (0%–15%, 0–750 mL) – Tachycardia
  - Grade 2 (15%–30%, 750–1500 mL) – Tachycardia, narrow pulse pressure, tachypnoea, anxiety
  - Grade 3 (30%–40%, 1500–2000 mL) – Tachycardia, tachypnoea, confusion, reduced urine output, reduced systolic blood pressure (BP)
  - Grade 4 (>40%, >2000 mL) – Tachycardia, coma, low urine output, unrecordable diastolic BP

What is the systemic inflammatory response syndrome (SIRS)? What can cause it?

- A systemic response to the inflammation of endothelium
- Defined by two or more of the following:
  - Temperature $\quad$ <36°C or >38°C
  - Heart rate (HR) $\quad$ >90/min
  - Respiratory rate (RR) $\quad$ >20/min or $PaCO_2$ <4.3 kPa
  - WCC $\quad$ >12 × 10^9/L or <4 × 10^9/L
- Causes include:
  - Injury (e.g. burns, trauma)
  - Inflammation (e.g. acute pancreatitis)
  - Infection (e.g. aspiration, faecal peritonitis)
  - Ischaemia (e.g. shock of any cause, reperfusion injury)
  - Iatrogenic (e.g. major surgery, blood transfusions)
  - Intoxication
  - Immune
  - Idiopathic

Distinguish SIRS from bacteraemia, sepsis, severe sepsis, septic shock and multi-organ dysfunction.

- *Bacteraemia* is the presence of bacteria in the blood as confirmed by microbiological culture.
- *Sepsis* is a systemic illness caused by microbial invasion of normally sterile body sites that is associated with one or more clinical signs. Sepsis is defined as SIRS plus documented evidence of infection.

- *Severe sepsis* is defined as sepsis associated with organ dysfunction, hypoperfusion abnormality or sepsis-induced hypotension.
- *Septic shock* is the presence of severe sepsis plus persistent or refractory hypotension or tissue hypoperfusion despite adequate intravenous (IV) fluid resuscitation.
- *Multi-organ dysfunction syndrome (or multi-organ failure)* is the presence of severe, acquired dysfunction of two or more organ systems in an acutely ill patient such that homeostasis cannot be maintained without intervention. Mortality is approximately 20% per involved organ system.

How would you manage a neutropaenic patient?

- A, B, C
- History – Malignancy, recent chemotherapy, immunosuppressants, human immunodeficiency virus (HIV), recent transfusion
- Physical examination – Signs of sepsis (fever, shock), peripheral/central vascular lines, systems review
- Septic screen – CXR, blood haematology and biochemistry, cultures (blood, sputum, urine, stool, wound swabs, cerebrospinal fluid [CSF])
- Commence broad spectrum in accordance with local guidelines and microbiologist advice
- Investigate source of infection – Further imaging, e.g. CT, bronchoscopy

PANCREATITIS

How would you manage a patient presenting with pancreatitis?

- A, B, C and fluid resuscitation
- History – Establish cause (gallstones, alcohol, trauma, steroids, mumps, autoimmune, hyperlipidaemia, hypercalcaemia, endoscopic retrograde cholangiopancreatography [ERCP], drugs, scorpion venom)
- Physical examination
- ABG – pO_2, acidotic
- Blood profile (full blood count [FBC], electrolytes, urea, LFTs, albumin, glucose)
- Ultrasound scan (USS) – To check for gallstones (may require urgent ERCP and sphincterotomy)
- Assess prognostic severity with, e.g. the Modified Glasgow (Imrie) Scoring (1 point for each criterion met on admission and again at 48 hours post admission. 1–2 points is associated with a mortality of <1%, 3–4 points with 15% and 6 points with a mortality approaching 100%).
- CT performed at 5–7 days post admission can demonstrate features of pancreatitis ranging from mild to severe, i.e. oedema, extra-pancreatic changes, fluid collection, necrosis.

What complications may arise?

- Mortality (approximately 10%)
- Local complications – Phlegmon, pseudocyst, abscess, ascites, haemorrhage, necrotizing pancreatitis, splenic vein thrombosis, fat necrosis
- Intestinal complications – Paralytic ileus, gastrointestinal haemorrhage
- Hepatobiliary complications – Jaundice, stricture of the common bile duct (CBD), portal vein thrombosis
- Systemic complications
  - Metabolic – Malnutrition, hypocalcaemia, hyperglycaemia, hypoalbuminaemia
  - Haematological – Disseminated intravascular coagulation (DIC)
  - Renal – Acute renal failure
  - Cardiovascular – Circulatory failure (shock), arrhythmias
  - Respiratory – Hypoxic acute respiratory failure (ARDS), pleural effusions

Modified Glasgow (Imrie) Scoring	
PO_2	<8 kPa (60 mmHg)
Age	>55
Neutr/WCC	$>15 \times 10^9$/L
Ca (corrected)	<2 mmol/L
Raised Ur	>16 mmol/L
Enzymes (LDH)	>600 IU/L
Albumin	<32 g/L
Sugar (glucose)	>10 mmol/L

RENAL FAILURE

What are the causes of acute renal failure following surgery?

- Pre-renal causes – Hypotension, hypovolaemia
- Renal causes – Nephrotoxic drugs (non-steroidal anti-inflammatory drugs [NSAIDs], gentamicin, angiotensin-converting-enzyme [ACE] inhibitors), sepsis, myoglobinuria, contrast media
- Post-renal causes – Blocked urinary catheter, ureteric injury, calculi, prostatic obstruction

What is the commonest cause of renal failure in surgical patients and why?

- Pre-renal failure
- Inadequate renal perfusion secondary to volume depletion

Where are the commonest surgical fluid losses?

- Haemorrhage
- Gastrointestinal
- Sepsis
- Third space

What is oliguria and how would you manage it?

- Urine output less than 0.5 mL/kg/hour
- Flush or change the urinary catheter
- Increase IV fluid filling if appearing fluid depleted but considering cardiac status
- More invasive monitoring, e.g. central venous pressure (CVP) line and 'fluid challenge'
- Consider diuretics but this may mask the underlying cause
- Check blood biochemistry – Electrolytes and urea e.g. hyperkalaemia, which may need treating
- Stop nephrotoxic drugs
- Treat sepsis aggressively
- Consider an abdominal USS to exclude hydronephrosis from obstructive uropathy
- If worsening renal function, increasing fluid retention and electrolyte disturbances, consider dialysis and discuss with ICU

ANALGESIA

How do you prescribe pain relief? What if the pain is still not controlled?

- World Health Organisation (WHO) Analgesic Ladder – Simple analgesics (paracetamol, NSAIDs), weak opiates (codeine, tramadol, co-codamol), strong opiates (morphine). Pethidine has been withdrawn from the latest edition of the WHO Guide.
- If not controlled, re-assess patient for worsening or new pathology. If inadequate analgesia, use additive approach as per WHO analgesic ladder.
- If still not controlled, discuss with pain team or anaesthetist for adjuncts or alternatives.

How may analgesics be given?

- Enteral
    - Oral (or via nasogastric [NG] tube, percutaneous endoscopic gastrostomy [PEG] etc.)
    - Rectal

- Parenteral
  - Intramuscular
  - IV
  - Subcutaneous (often used in palliative care, e.g. syringe drivers)
  - Transdermal (e.g. fentanyl patches)
  - Epidural
  - Intrathecal
  - Local anaesthetic field blocks

What is patient-controlled analgesia and what are its benefits?

- The patient presses a button that delivers a prescribed dose of IV or epidural analgesia, at preset intervals from an electronically controlled infusion pump.
- Faster pain-sensation to pain-relief time and better pain control.
- Objective measure of how much analgesia required over time.
- Reduced nursing input and medication errors.
- Has an internal safety mechanism to prevent opioid overdose because of the 'lock out' time period. If the patient administers too much they fall asleep and stop pressing the button.

PRE-OPERATIVE ASSESSMENT

How would you assess a patient's fitness for surgery?

- History – Previous surgery/anaesthetic, Intensive Treatment Unit (ITU) admission, exercise tolerance, medication, smoker, respiratory symptoms
- Physical examination – Cardiorespiratory signs (wheeze, cough, dyspnoea, heart murmur, dysrhythmia)
- ECG, CXR
- Blood profile – Haematology (anaemia, infection), coagulation, biochemistry (renal function)
- Additional investigations
  - ABG
  - Lung spirometry (peak expiratory flow rate [PEFR], FEV_1, forced vital capacity [FVC])
  - ECHO
  - Exercise tolerance test
- You should be aware that the National Institute for Health and Clinical Excellence (NICE) has produced guidelines on what pre-operative investigations are required for individual groups of patients. Recommendations are based on the age of the patient, the American Society of Anesthesiologists (ASA) grade of patient and the type of surgery.

What do you do if you are concerned regarding a patient's fitness for surgery?

- Early discussion with the anaesthetist performing the list.
- Arrange appropriate specialist consults early with respect to the areas of concern, specifically asking for approval for surgery.
- If necessary delay the surgical procedure until it is safe to proceed, unless it is an emergency and the risk is outweighed by the gain.
- Inform the operating team and bookings office early regarding possible delays to the surgical procedure.

JAUNDICE

What specific questions would you ask a jaundiced patient and why?

- Presence of pain – Painless jaundice may suggest malignancy
- Presence of pale stools and/or dark urine, pruritus – Suggests obstruction of the biliary tree, e.g. gallstone, tumour
- Unintentional weight loss – Suggests a possible malignancy obstructing the biliary tree, e.g. head of pancreas carcinoma, cholangiocarcinoma
- Foreign travel and/or ingested shell fish – Suggests viral hepatitis A
- Recent transfusions – Suggests haemolytic anaemia or infective hepatitis
- Family history of jaundice – Hereditary conditions (e.g. Crigler–Najjar syndrome)
- Current medications – Hepatotoxic drugs
- Alcohol intake – Alcoholic hepatitis, cirrhosis
- IV drug abuse and sexual history – Infective hepatitis

What are the causes of jaundice?

- Pre-hepatic causes
  - Haemolysis
  - Gilbert's syndrome and other congenital enzymatic defects in bilirubin metabolism (e.g. Crigler–Najjar syndrome)
  - Dyserythropoiesis
- Hepatocellular causes (cirrhosis)
  - Congenital/genetic – Haemochromatosis, Wilson's, α1-antitrypsin deficiency
  - Alcohol
  - Drugs and toxins
  - Autoimmune, e.g. primary biliary cirrhosis
  - Infections – Viral hepatitis, leptospirosis, cytomegalovirus (CMV), HIV, Epstein–Barr virus (EBV) etc.
  - Neoplasia – Primary (hepatocellular carcinoma) and secondary/metastatic
  - Cardiac cirrhosis – CCF
- Post-hepatic (obstructive) jaundice
  - Gallstones within the CBD
  - Carcinoma of the head of pancreas

- Ascending cholangitis
- Carcinoma around the ampulla of Vater
- Lymphadenopathy at the porta hepatis
- Primary sclerosing cholangitis
- Mirizzi's syndrome
- Benign strictures of the CBD
  - Inflammatory (pancreatitis)
  - Post-operative
  - Post-radiotherapy
- Malignant strictures of the CBD (cholangiocarcinoma)
- Congenital – Biliary atresia

If you suspect a patient has obstructive jaundice, how would you proceed and why?

- A, B, C
- History – As above
- Physical examination – Pyrexia, tenderness in right upper quadrant (RUQ), palpable mass or nodes, palpable gallbladder (Courvoisier's law), urine dipstick, stool sample
- Blood profile – Haematology (anaemia, inflammation – cholecystitis/cholangitis), biochemistry (hydration status, hepatorenal syndrome), liver function tests (alanine transaminase [ALT], aspartate aminotransferase [AST], Alk phos, bilirubin, albumin – hepatitic/obstructive picture), coagulation (derangement secondary to liver dysfunction needs correction prior to intervention)
- Blood cultures – If suspect cholangitis
- USS – Cholecystitis/cholangitis, gallstones, dilated CBD, head of pancreas tumour, cholangiocarcinoma, hepatitis

How would your subsequent management differ following a USS report of an obstructing gallstone from a report of an obstructing tumour mass?

- Gallstones – Consider urgent ERCP and sphincterotomy to remove the obstructing gallstone.
- Tumour – Requires urgent CT staging and multidisciplinary team (MDT) discussion for subsequent therapy. However, in worsening obstructive jaundice, immediate biliary drainage and stenting may be required initially. This can be performed percutaneously under radiological guidance.

What are the complications of surgery in the jaundiced patient?

- Altered fluid balance – Hypoalbuminaemia (leading to peripheral oedema and ascites), secondary hyperaldosteronism (leading to sodium retention and hypokalaemia)
- Acid–base disturbances
- Coagulopathy
- Hepatorenal syndrome (leading to renal failure)

- Altered drug metabolism
- Metabolic derangements, e.g. hypoglycaemia
- Increased risk of sepsis
- Delayed wound healing
- Malnutrition
- Hepatic encephalopathy
- Increased risk to hospital staff (if infective hepatitis)

TRAUMA

How would you manage a patient brought in from a road traffic accident who is tachycardic?

- A, B, C, cervical spine control, fluid resuscitation
- Glasgow coma scale (GCS)
- History
- Physical examination – Assess injuries (head, chest, abdomen, pelvis, limbs)
- Trauma x-ray series – C-spine, CXR, pelvis
- Blood profile – Haematology, biochemistry, group and save or X-match
- Catheterise for monitoring of fluid balance, if appropriate
- If indicated – CT, laparotomy

How might you gain venous access?

- Peripheral – Antecubital, forearm, saphenous veins
- Peripheral venous cut down – Great saphenous vein
- Central – Femoral, subclavian, internal jugular veins (Seldinger technique)

Shortly after central venous line insertion, the patient becomes hypoxic, tachypnoeic and tachycardic. What might be the cause?

- Pneumothorax
- Haemothorax
- Air embolism
- Causes unrelated to central venous line insertion – Fat embolus, ARDS

If the patient arrests, what may be the cause? What would you then do?

- Tension pneumothorax.
- Insert a large bore cannula into the second intercostal space, mid-clavicular line on the side of the suspected pneumothorax. (A chest drain will then be required for definitive management.)
- Other reversible causes of cardiac arrest – Cardiac tamponade, thromboembolism, toxins, hypoxia, hypovolaemia, hyper/hypokalaemia, hypothermia (remember the 4T's and 4H's).

ACUTE RESPIRATORY DISTRESS SYNDROME

A surgical patient develops hypoxaemia with minimal improvement on supplementary oxygen therapy. You request a CXR (Figure 5.3) which shows signs of pulmonary oedema but there are no other clinical signs of heart failure. What is the likely diagnosis?

- ARDS (non-cardiogenic pulmonary oedema)

What is ARDS?

- Severe acute lung injury
- Progressive and refractory hypoxaemia
- Diffuse bilateral pulmonary infiltrates on CXR
- Non-cardiac cause (normal pulmonary artery wedge pressure ≤ 18 mmHg)
- Reduced lung compliance
- Ventilation–perfusion mismatch

What might be causing it?

- Direct (pulmonary)
  - Pneumonia
  - Chest trauma
  - Aspiration pneumonitis
  - Near-drowning
  - Inhalational injury

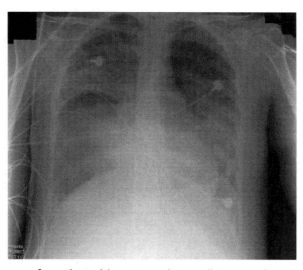

Figure 5.3 Chest x-ray of a patient with acute respiratory distress syndrome.

- Indirect (systemic)
  - Sepsis
  - Shock
  - Burns
  - Polytrauma
  - Head injury
  - Embolus (fat, air)
  - Acute pancreatitis
  - Cardiopulmonary bypass
  - Transfusion

How are you going to manage this patient?

- A, B, C
- History and physical examination
- Investigate cause
- Oxygen therapy
- Early discussion with anaesthetist and chest physiotherapist regarding ventilatory support

What type of respiratory failure would you expect to see? Why?

- Type 1 respiratory failure (stiff lungs in ARDS causes problems with gas exchange, resulting in hypoxia. There may be compensatory hyperventilation which may lead to hypocarbia).
- In Type 2 respiratory failure, there is a ventilatory problem causing hypoventilation and resulting in hypercarbia as well as hypoxia. Surgical causes include head injury, stroke, respiratory depressants, trauma, epidural anaesthesia, tumour etc. Other causes include COPD, asthma etc.

How do you manage ARDS?

- Treat cause and support patient
- Intubation, high FiO_2
- Low tidal volumes, avoiding barotrauma
- 'Permissive hypercapnia' to prevent barotrauma and volutrauma
- Pressure-controlled, inverse inspiratory – Expiratory ratio ventilation
- PEEP/CPAP
- Prone ventilation
- Physiotherapy
- Keep lungs dry, use inotropes to support cardiac output (CO)
- Treat sepsis
- Nutritional support
- Treat complications early
- Steroids may prevent progression to the destructive fibrotic phase of the disease
- Consider NO, prostacyclin, surfactant

FLUID BALANCE

How do you tell if a patient is dehydrated? How would you resuscitate them?

- Dry mucous membranes, tachycardia, reduced urine output, drowsy etc.
- IV dextrose (mostly moves into cells to rehydrate)

How would you resuscitate a shocked, hypovolaemic patient?

- Colloid, blood (fluid volume is retained in the vascular compartment)
- Hartmann's solution (maintains composition of extracellular fluid [ECF] when large volumes of resuscitation fluid are given)

Which fluids are good for maintenance?

- 0.9% normal saline with potassium supplementation
- Hartmann's solution

Which factors determine how much fluid should be given?

- Pre-existing fluid deficit
- **Maintenance fluids required**
  - Ongoing losses (sensible and insensible losses)

Which surgical patients require increased maintenance fluids?

- Pyrexial
- Ileus
- Vomiting
- High stoma output
- Fistulae
- Pancreatitis
- Polyuric (common in neurosurgical patients)

What options do you have to monitor fluid balance status?

- History – Feels thirsty
- Physical examination – Mucous membranes, skin turgor, GCS, HR, BP, jugular venous pulse (JVP), urine output (minimum 0.5 mL/kg/hour), pulse oximetry
- Blood profile – Renal function, haematocrit
- Urine output, urine specific gravity
- ECG, CXR
- CVPs
- Pulmonary artery flotation catheter – Monitors left heart pressures and CO

What information can you gain from the pulse oximeter? Is it reliable?

- HR, arterial oxygen saturation, peripheral perfusion status
- Not reliable if – Saturation <70%, patient moving, venous congestion, coloured nail varnish

BOWEL OBSTRUCTION

A patient presents to A&E post-laparotomy with vomiting, absolute constipation and abdominal pain. What is the likely diagnosis? How would you confirm it? What is the most common aetiology?

- Small-bowel obstruction
- Abdominal x-ray (AXR) – Central dilated loops (>3 cm diameter), valvulae conniventes
- Adhesions. Other causes include hernia, strictures (e.g. Crohn's), tumours, gallstones etc.

How would you manage this patient?

- A, B, C and fluid resuscitation
- History and physical examination
- Nil by mouth (NBM) and NG tube
- Catheterise
- IV fluids (Hartmann's or normal saline with potassium supplementation)
- Analgesia and anti-emetics

What are common causes of large-bowel obstruction? How would you investigate it?

- Tumours, strictures
- AXR, CT staging
- Contrast enema (barium/gastrograffin)
- MR staging for cancers of the rectum

What problems can arise with patients on total parenteral nutrition (TPN)?

- Line sepsis
- Pneumothorax
- Infective endocarditis
- Metabolic disturbances
- Refeeding syndrome

TRANSFUSION

A patient has suffered major trauma and requires a massive transfusion. Which type of packed red blood cell product can be given to a patient with blood group AB?

- Any type – group AB = universal acceptor
- Group O neg = universal donor

What is the volume of 1 unit of packed red cells? How does transfusing 1 unit affect the Hb concentration?

- Approximately 300 mL
- Dose of 4 mL/kg (one pack to 70 kg adult) typically raises venous Hb concentration by about 1 g/dL

Are there any potential problems that may arise, post-transfusion?

- Immune reactions – Haemolysis
- Volume overload
- Coagulopathy – Absence of clotting factors especially factor V and VIII (thus supplement with fresh frozen plasma [FFP])
- Thrombocytopenia
- Hyperkalaemia – Potassium leaks from packed red cells during storage
- Hypocalcaemia – Citrate is added to the packed red cell suspension to increase longevity during storage but this chelates calcium
- Hypothermia – Packed red cell blood is stored at 4°C. N.B. shelf-life of packed red cell blood = 35 days at 4°C
- Infection – Hepatitis B virus (HBV), hepatitis C virus (HCV), Syphilis, *Yersinia*, *Staphylococcus*

You are called to see a patient being transfused who is complaining of a headache and abdominal pain and is now pyrexial and has started to drop their BP. What is the diagnosis? How do you manage this patient?

- Haemolytic transfusion reaction
- Stop the transfusion
- A, B, C and fluid resuscitation
- Blood profile – Haematology (anaemia secondary to haemolysis), biochemistry (bilirubin)
- Repeat group and save, and cross-match (Coombs' testing)
- Send blood cultures in case of sepsis from contaminated blood. History and physical examination

DRUGS

What might you do to improve the circulation status of a patient in septic shock? Why?

- Fluid resuscitation – Pyrexia, with increased fluid losses through sweat.
- Inotropic agents – There is a hyperdynamic circulation with peripheral vasodilatation.

What are inotropic agents? Name a few examples.

- Drugs that act on alpha- and beta-adrenergic receptors causing increase in cardiac contractility and rate, and increase in peripheral vascular resistance. This therefore improves CO and BP.
- Dopamine, dobutamine, adrenaline, noradrenaline.

What sedative drugs do you know? How would you reverse their effects?

- Benzodiazepines (e.g. midazolam) – Flumazenil
- Barbiturates (e.g. thiopentone) – No known antidote, respiratory support
- IV anaesthetic agents (e.g. propofol) – No known antidote but short duration of action
- Inhalational anaesthetic agents (e.g. isoflurane) – Pure oxygen

What types of muscle relaxants do you know? Give examples.

- Depolarising agents – Suxamethonium
- Non-depolarising agents – Vecuronium, atracurium, rocuronium (reversed by neostigmine, or newer agents such as sugammadex)

HEAD INJURY

A patient complains of headache, nausea and is drowsy after a head injury. Is this significant? Why? What would you do next?

- Yes
- Possible raised intracranial pressure and danger of reduced cerebral perfusion pressure and cerebral herniation (Monro–Kellie doctrine of fixed intracranial space)
- History and physical examination
- GCS – Intubate early if clinical picture suggests deterioration to 8/15 or less
- Check for papilloedema
- Full neurological examination
- CT head

What might cause raised increased intracranial pressure (ICP)?

- Intracranial bleeding
- Brain tumours
- Cerebral oedema
- Hydrocephalus

Name some secondary causes of brain injury.

- Primary brain injury takes places when the primary insult occurs and is considered irreversible. Secondary brain injury results from processes initiated by the primary insult that occur some time later and that may be prevented or ameliorated. Management of head injury aims to prevent secondary brain injury. Causes of secondary brain injury include
  - Raised intracranial pressure
  - Vasospasm
  - Hypoxia
  - Hypotension
  - Hypercarbia
  - Hyperpyrexia
  - Hyponatraemia and other electrolyte disturbances
  - Hyperglycaemia/hypoglycaemia
  - Anaemia
  - Sepsis
  - Raised venous pressure
  - Seizures

What do you understand by the Monro-Kelly hypothesis, or doctrine?

- This describes the pressure-volume relationship between intracranial pressure, CSF, blood and brain. The hypothesis states that the cranial compartment is incompressible and therefore the volume inside the cranium is fixed. Its constituents (brain, blood, CSF) create an equilibrium such that any increase in volume of one must be compensated by a decrease in volume of another (Figure 5.4). For example, an increase in lesion volume (e.g. intracerebral haemorrhage or tumour) will be compensated for by a downward displacement of CSF and venous blood. These compensatory mechanisms are able to maintain normal ICP for any change in volume less than approximately 100-120 mL. When this mechanism has no further reserve capacity, the intracranial pressure increases rapidly. The result is hypoperfusion and herniation (Figure 5.5).

How can the ICP be reduced?

- Patient positioning – Nursing the patient head up
- Avoid obstruction of venous drainage from the head (making sure C-spine immobilisation collar is not too tight)
- Adjusting $PaCO_2$ by manipulating ventilation – Adjusts intracranial vessel vasoconstriction/dilatation
- Fluid balance, e.g. diuretics, mannitol etc.
- Sedation (e.g. barbiturates), with or without muscle relaxants
- Steroids (e.g. dexamethasone) can reduce cerebral oedema around tumours
- Induced hypothermia and anticonvulsants (lower metabolic demands of brain tissue)

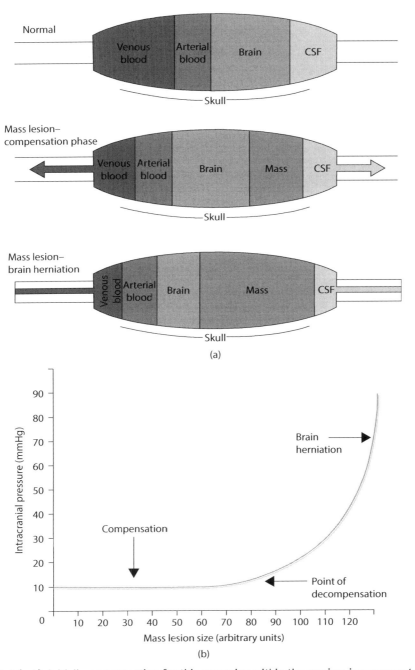

Figure 5.4 (a, b) Initially, compensation for this expansion within the cranium is compensated for by displacement of CSF and venous blood. When this mechanism has no further reserve capacity, the intracranial pressure increases rapidly. The result is hypoperfusion and herniation.

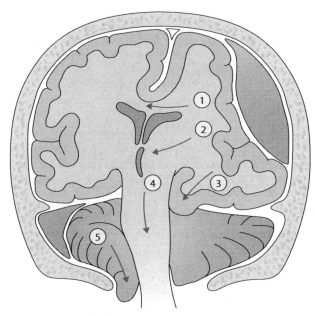

Figure 5.5 Brain herniation. Herniation of the cingulate gyrus under the falx cerebri is called 'subfalcine herniation'. (1) Herniation is associated with midline shift. (2) Herniation of the uncus of the temporal lobe (3) is associated with compression of the ipsilateral third nerve. Central herniation (4) and tonsillar herniation (5) are associated with compression of brainstem structures.

- Tapping off CSF via a ventricular catheter
- Emergency surgical evacuation of any haematoma causing mass effect (burr holes, craniotomy, decompressive craniectomy)

What emergency neurosurgical procedures may be undertaken for head injury?

- Burr hole
  - Frontal
  - Parietal
  - Temporal
  - Occipital
- Craniotomy/craniectomy
- Ventricular tap
  - Frontal burr hole
- Elevation of compound depressed skull facture

What are the indications for CT in head injuries?

- Falling GCS
- Persisting neurological signs, headache or vomiting post-resuscitation
- Clinical suspicion of a fracture of the skull base – CSF rhinorrhoea/otorrhoea, Battle's sign, subconjunctival haemorrhage with no ascertainable posterior border

- Suspected penetrating head injury
- Post-traumatic seizures
- Patient has a coagulopathy (e.g. on warfarin).
- The patient is difficult to fully assess (e.g. alcohol intoxication).

What are the intracranial abnormalities that indicate urgent neurosurgical management?

- High or mixed density intracranial lesion (size and site)
- Midline shift
- Obliteration of third ventricle/basal cisterns
- Contra-lateral ventricular dilatation
- Intracranial air
- Subarachnoid or intraventricular haemorrhage

BRAINSTEM DEATH

You are the ST2 in general surgery and you get called at 2 AM by the ST3 in ICU saying that your surgical patient is now brainstem dead. You go to ICU to review the case. Between the ICU ST3 and yourself, can you confirm brainstem death?

- No.
- Can only be legally confirmed by two clinicians, one of whom is a consultant and the other General Medical Council (GMC) registered for at least 5 years. They must also be either an intensivist, anaesthetist, neurologist or neurosurgeon.

What are the clinical criteria for brainstem death?

- Patient in an apnoeic coma (reliant entirely on mechanical ventilation due to the complete absence of spontaneous ventilation) with a GCS of 3/15
- Identification of the cause of apnoeic coma
- Exclusion of reversible causes (drugs, alcohol, hypothyroidism, uraemia, hypoglycaemia, hypothermia etc.)
- Clinical demonstration of absence of brainstem reflexes.
  - Absent pupillary light reflex
  - Absent corneal reflex
  - Absent gag and cough reflex
  - Absent vestibulo-ocular reflex (caloric testing)
  - Absent oculo-cephalic reflexes (doll's eye manoeuvre)
  - Absent cranial motor function
  - Absent respiratory drive following a rise in $PaCO_2$ (apnoea testing)

You get a call from the organ transplantation team confirming that the patient is legally registered for organ donation. They ask you if the patient's clinical condition meets the criteria for donation. What do they mean?

- Confirmation of brainstem death
- No sepsis
- No history of malignancy (except for brain tumours)
- No history if IV drug abuse
- HIV and HBV negative
- No history of MI (for heart donation)
- No history of alcohol abuse (for liver donation)

Which organs may be donated?

- Heart
- Lungs
- Liver
- Kidneys
- Pancreas
- Small bowel
- Bone
- Tendon
- Cornea
- Skin

CHAPTER 6: HEAD AND NECK

DYSPHAGIA: HISTORY TAKING

You are a junior doctor on Mr Smith's general surgery team. Mr Smith has asked you to clerk a new patient in the outpatient clinic. The GP referral letter is attached. After you have taken the history you will be asked to present it to one of the examiners as though she or he were the consultant. She or he will then ask you for your differential diagnosis, what signs you would look for on examination and what investigations you would request?

Take a standard focused surgical history (presenting complaint, history presenting complaint, past medical history, drug history and allergies, social history, family history, systemic enquiry), but in particular enquire about the following:

- Duration
- Time course and progression
- Level of food 'sticking' – Back throat, thyroid cartilage, suprasternal notch, retrosternal
- Difficulty with solids, liquids or both
- Problems swallowing own saliva (absolute dysphagia)
- Intermittent or continuous. The former implies a neurological problem or achalasia
- Odynophagia (painful swallowing)
- Referred otalgia (a fairly specific symptom of malignancy)
- Dysphonia
- Risk factors – Smoking and alcohol
- Weight loss
- Regurgitation, coughing at night, halitosis, waterbrash, indigestion, heartburn, acid reflux, chest infections
- Neurological symptoms (e.g. muscle weakness, fatigability) and history of neurological disease

---

Drs G Jones and S Williams

17 High Street
London

The Consultant Surgeon
St Mary's Hospital
London

Re: Harry Green, 69 Grey Lane, Middlesex

Dear Doctor

This 60-year-old patient rarely comes to the surgery, but he came today complaining of difficulty in swallowing.

Best wishes

Yours sincerely
Simon Williams

Differential diagnosis

Lesions of the mouth/pharynx:

- Recurrent aphthous ulcers
- Stomatitis/glossitis/tonsillitis
- Quinsy/retropharyngeal abscess

Intraluminal:

- Foreign body
- Polypoid tumours

Intramural:

- Peptic stricture (gastro-oesophageal reflux disease)
- Carcinoma oesophagus/gastric cardia
- Infective (cytomegalovirus [CMV], herpes simplex virus (HSV), human immunodeficiency virus [HIV], Candida)
- Stricture secondary to ingestion caustic substances and radiotherapy
- Pharyngeal/oesophageal web (Plummer–Vinson or George–Paterson–Brown–Kelly syndrome)
- Schatzki's (lower oesophageal) ring
- Pharyngeal pouch

Extrinsic compression:

- Goitre with retrosternal extension
- Para-oesophageal (rolling) hiatus hernia
- Mediastinal tumours
- Enlarged lymph nodes
- Left atrial enlargement (mitral stenosis)
- 'Dysphagia lusoria' (compression from abnormally placed great vessels)

Motility disorders:

- Following cardiovascular accident (CVA) (stroke)
- Achalasia
- Diffuse oesophageal spasm
- Scleroderma (part of the CREST syndrome)
- Parkinson's disease (hence sialorrhoea)
- Bulbar/pseudobulbar palsy
- Myasthenia gravis
- Motor neurone disease
- Hysteria (globus hystericus)

Signs to look for on examination:

- General physical status of patient (cachexia, JACCOL – Jaundice, anaemia, cyanosis, clubbing, oedema, lymphadenopathy)
- Check for peripheral stigmata of gastrointestinal disease such as koilonychia, angular cheilitis and glossitis (Plummer–Vinson syndrome) or features of the CREST syndrome
- Neck examination, noting the presence of any neck lumps (e.g. pharyngeal pouch) and checking for cervical lymphadenopathy and supraclavicular lymphadenopathy – Virchow's node (Troisier's sign)

- Abdominal examination checking for masses, ascites, hepato-splenomegaly
- Neurological examination – A variety of neurological abnormalities will be associated with dysphagia of neuromuscular origin
- A full Ear, Nose and Throat (ENT) examination including fibre-optic laryngoscopy

Investigations

Blood tests:

- Haematology – Full blood count (FBC), iron studies, erythrocyte sedimentation rate (ESR)
  - Anaemia (Malignancy, Plummer–Vinson)
  - Serum iron/total iron binding capacity (TIBC)/ferritin (Plummer–Vinson, gastrointestinal [GI] bleed)
  - ESR (malignancy, scleroderma)
- Biochemistry
  - U+Es (dehydration)
  - Liver function tests (LFTs) (liver metastases)
- Immunology
  - Autoantibody screen (scleroderma)

Radiology:

- Chest x-ray (CXR) (anterior-posterior [AP] and lateral)
  - Thyroid goitre extension, left atrial enlargement, tumours, foreign body, aspiration, achalasia (air-fluid level behind heart), thoracic aortic aneurysm
- Barium swallow (in the absence of absolute dysphagia otherwise there is a risk of aspiration)
  - Motility disorder (e.g. achalasia), pharyngeal pouch (oesophago-gastro-duodenoscopy [OGD] risks perforation), benign/malignant stricture, external compression, reflux
- Computed tomography (CT) thorax
  - Staging of tumour

OGD (±biopsy and *Helicobacter pylori* status):

- Diagnostic
  - Malignant stricture (tumour), benign peptic stricture, oesophagitis (inflammatory/infective), achalasia, foreign body
- Therapeutic
  - Balloon dilatation
- Surveillance
  - Barrett's oesophagus (pre-malignant)

Specific investigations:

- Oesophageal endoluminal ultrasound scan (USS) (staging oesophageal carcinoma)
- Bronchoscopy/mediastinoscopy (assessment of invasion of oesophageal carcinoma)

- Liver USS (staging carcinoma)
- Laparoscopy (staging carcinoma)
- Oesophageal manometry (oesophageal spasm)
- 24-hour oesophageal pH monitoring (oesophageal reflux)

LUMP IN THE NECK: HISTORY TAKING

You are a junior doctor on Mr Jones' ENT team. Mr Jones has asked you to clerk a new patient in the outpatient clinic. The GP referral letter is attached. After you have taken the history, you will be asked to present it to one of the examiners as though she or he were the consultant.

Drs S Green and H. Brown

---

1 Grange Road
London

The Consultant ENT Surgeon
St Peter's Hospital
Edinburgh

Re: George Latimer, 16 Kings Road, London

Dear Doctor

I would be grateful if you could see this 70-year-old gentleman who came to us with a lump in the neck.

Best wishes

Yours sincerely

Dr H Brown

Take a standard focused surgical history (presenting complaint, history presenting complaint, past medical history, drug history and allergies, social history, family history, systemic enquiry), but in particular enquire about the following:

- Age
- Site of lump
- Single or multiple
- Onset, duration and developmental time course (congenital vs. acquired)
- Presence or absence of pain
- Associated symptoms (dysphagia, dysphonia, odynophagia, referred otalgia, globus sensation, cough, haemoptysis, weight loss, symptoms of thyroid dysfunction, sore throats, intraoral diseases such as tooth decay)

- Personal habits/risk factors (smoking, alcohol, betel nuts etc.)
- Previous radiation or surgery
- Systemic symptoms – Fever, night sweats, pruritus, anorexia, malaise
- Family history and tuberculosis (TB) contacts
- Foreign travel and risk factors for HIV infection

LUMP IN THE NECK: EXAMINATION

The same approach can also be used for any skin lesion in the head and neck region.

On entering the room:

- Introduce yourself to the patient (permission)
- Obtain consent
- Obtain adequate exposure (position)
- Check if the patient has any pain (pain)
- Wash hands

Inspection

After determining the number of lumps, apply the rule of S's:

1. Site (anatomical triangle neck or level in the neck)
   - The borders of the anterior triangle are the anterior border of the sternocleidomastoid muscle, the ramus of the mandible and the midline. The borders of the posterior triangle are the posterior border of sternocleidomastoid, the middle one-third of the clavicle and the anterior border of the trapezius muscle.
   - An alternative approach is to state which level of the neck the lump is situated in, according to the Memorial Sloan–Kettering classification (Figure 6.1):
     - Level 1 = Submental (Ia) and submandibular (Ib) areas
     - Level 2 = Upper third sternocleidomastoid
     - Level 3 = Middle third sternocleidomastoid
     - Level 4 = Lower third sternocleidomastoid
     - Level 5 = Posterior triangle
     - Level 6 = Pretracheal and prelaryngeal areas

2. Size (A × B cm)

3. Shape (hemispherical, lobulated etc.)

4. Surface and smoothness – Overlying punctum, smooth/bosselated surface

5. Skin overlying the lump – Skin changes, skin colour, scars (taking care not to miss any faint tracheostomy or thyroidectomy scars), evidence of previous radiotherapy

6. Surroundings – Other lumps, satellite nodules

7. Special characteristics – E.g. moves with swallowing, protrusion of tongue, pulsatile etc.

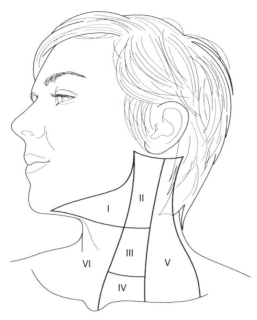

Figure 6.1 Oncological levels in the neck.

Palpation

1. Tenderness – Before touching the lump, check with the patient first whether it is tender

2. Temperature – Using the back of the hand (which is more sensitive)

3. Consistency – Soft, firm, hard, bony hard

4. Edge – Diffuse or defined

5. Fluctuance – In two planes at right angles to each other (Paget's sign)

6. Try to ascertain which layer the lump is in

To determine its relationship to the skin, ask if you can pinch the skin overlying the lump or if you can move the skin over it. If either of these is the case, the lump lies deep in the skin. Alternatively, if the lump moves with the skin, it lies within the skin.

For skin lesions, ask is it flush with the skin, or raised?

To determine the relationship of the lump to underlying muscles (e.g. sternocleidomastoid), ask the patient to tense/contract the muscle:

- Test for mobility/fixity of the lump at rest in two orthogonal planes.
- Then ask the patient to contract the underlying muscle.
- Ask yourself is the lump more or less prominent?
- Ask yourself is the lump more or less mobile with the muscle contracted (in two planes)?

Insider's Tip

As a general rule, if the lump
- Retains mobility and is more prominent when underlying muscle is contracted = *Lump is superficial to muscle.*
- Is more prominent but less mobile when underlying muscle is contracted = *Lump is attached to fascia or superficial surface of muscle.*
- Is less mobile and less prominent when underlying muscle is contracted = *Lump is within muscle.*
- Is less mobile and less prominent when underlying muscle is contracted = *Lump is deep to muscle.*

The one exception to the rule occurs when there is a *defect* in the muscle. In such cases, although the lump arises in, or deep, to the muscle, it appears more prominent when the muscle is contracted (e.g. ruptured muscle fibres as in a torn long head of biceps, incisional hernias, divarication of the rectus sheath etc.).

---

7. Never forget to assess the regional lymph node status.

8. Extra tests (if indicated) – Pulsatility, compressibility, thrill, transillumination, expansility, cough impulse, reducibility.

9. Palpate the normal structures of the neck – The hyoid bone, thyroid prominence of laryngeal cartilage, laryngeal cartilage, cricoid cartilage and trachea. Gently displace the larynx from side to side and feel for the normal laryngeal crepitus as the laryngeal cartilaginous framework is moved over the prevertebral muscle and fascia (this is lost in postcricoid tumours and in retropharyngeal abscesses; Trotter's sign).

Percussion

May be useful in defining if a goitre has retrosternal extension.

Auscultation

Bruits (e.g. Graves' goitre, carotid artery aneurysm, chemodectoma etc.)

Thank the patient and wash hands.

Summarise and offer your differential diagnosis.

Note:

If the case is cervical lymphadenopathy, do not forget to check the drainage sites (Figure 6.2). This will necessitate a complete ENT examination including examination of the postnasal space, oral cavity, oropharynx and fibre-optic laryngoscopy. In addition, offer to check other sites for lymphadenopathy (axilla, epitrochlear and inguinal regions, spleen, liver etc.), which may become involved, for instance in lymphoma and infections such as Epstein–Barr virus (EBV).

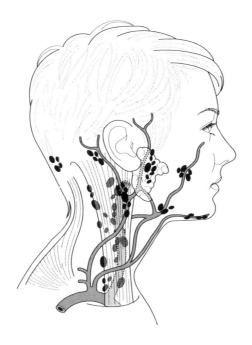

Figure 6.2 Lymphatic drainage and distribution.

NECK SWELLINGS: DIFFERENTIAL DIAGNOSIS

Midline neck swelling	Lateral neck swelling
• Sebaceous cyst	• Sebaceous cyst
• Lipoma	• Lipoma
• Thyroglossal duct cyst	• Cervical lymph node
• Solitary nodule of thyroid isthmus	• Thyroid gland enlargement
• Pyramidal thyroid lobe	• Branchial cyst
• Dermoid cyst	• Carotid body tumour
• Subhyoid bursae	• Pharyngeal pouch
• Plunging ranula	• Cystic hygroma
• Pretracheal, prelaryngeal (level VI) lymph node	
• Chondroma of the thyroid cartilage or larynx	

Multiple lumps

- Lymph nodes (invariably)
- Cold abscess (TB, actinomycosis)

Single Lumps

Superficial

- Sebaceous cyst
- Lipoma
- Dermoid cyst
- Abscess

Deep

	Anterior triangle	Posterior triangle
Does not move with swallowing	• Submandibular swelling • Parotid swelling • Branchial cyst • Carotid body tumour • Carotid artery aneurysm • Sternomastoid 'tumour' • Lymph node/cold abscess • Laryngocele chondroma	• Cystic hygroma (lymphangioma) • Pharyngeal pouch • Cervical rib • Subclavian artery aneurysm • Tumour of clavicle • Lymph node/cold abscess
Moves with swallowing	• Thyroglossal duct cyst • Thyroid gland • Thyroid isthmus lymph node	

If you are asked how you would manage any neck lump, the answer is always **triple assessment**, namely:

- History and clinical examination
- Imaging (USS/CT/MRI/Radionucleotide scan)
- Fine-needle aspiration cytology/biopsy

THYROID STATUS: HISTORY TAKING

Local pressure symptoms:

- Neck lumps – Duration, change in size with time etc.
- Pain
- Dysphagia

- Stridor/dyspnoea
- Hoarseness
- Cosmesis

Questions about thyroid status:

- Are you taking any medications?
- Have you had any thyroid operations, or radioiodine treatments, in the past?
- Are you affected by temperature? Do you prefer hot or cold?
- Have you lost or gained weight?
- Do you have constipation or diarrhoea?
- How is your appetite?
- Do you get palpitations?
- Have your periods changed?
- Have you noticed any change in your appearance/face?
- Have you become more anxious?
- Has your skin/hair changed?
- Do you have any problems with your eyes? (protruding eyes, difficulty closing eyelids, pain (secondary to exposure keratitis), double vision)

THYROID STATUS: EXAMINATION

On entering the room:

- Introduce yourself to the patient (permission)
- Obtain consent
- Obtain adequate exposure (position)
- Check if the patient has any pain (pain)
- Wash hands

Inspection

Perform a **General Survey**:

- Observe the patient's demeanour – Are they anxious and fidgety suggesting thyrotoxicosis, or are they slow and lethargic suggesting hypothyroidism? Is the patient thin or fat?

Palpation

Look in the **hands** for:

- Fine tremor (place a piece of paper on the patient's outstretched arms, palms facing down and the fingers extended and separated)
- Thyroid acropachy (a form of nail clubbing)

- Onycholysis (separation of the nail from the nail bed)
- Palmar erythema
- Warm, moist, sweaty palms
- Pulse (tachycardia, atrial fibrillation)
- Vitiligo

Look at the eyes for:

- Lid retraction (upper lid higher than normal, lower lid in correct position) (Figure 6.3).
- Lid lag – Gently restrain the patient's head to prevent movement and ask the patient to follow your finger with their eyes as you lower it slowly from above. Do **not** do this in a rapid fashion. Lid lag occurs when the upper lid does not keep pace with the eyeball and occurs because of spasm of the smooth muscle in the upper eyelid secondary to increased sympathetic tone in thyrotoxicosis.
- Proptosis/exophthalmos (look from in front, the side and from above; the sclera is visible below or all around the iris).
- Chemosis.
- Ophthalmoplegia (eye movements).
- Optic nerve involvement (visual acuity).
- Look in the **mouth** for a lingual thyroid
- Examine the **thyroid** gland itself
- Examine the **legs**
- Check reflexes and look for evidence of pretibial myxoedema
- Ask the patient to stand up with their arms across their chest

  - Look for proximal myopathy which can occur in hypothyroidism or hyperthyroidism

Thank the patient and wash hands.

Summarise and offer your differential diagnosis.

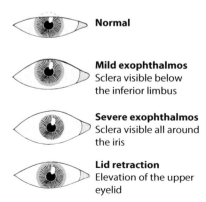

Figure 6.3 Exophthalmos versus lid retraction.

Assessment of thyroid status

	Hyperthyroid	Hypothyroid
General	Restlessness, anxiety, weight loss, intolerance to heat	Dull, mental lethargy, intolerance to cold, brittle hair
Hands	Nails (acropachy, onycholysis), palms (sweaty, warm, palmar erythema), fine tremor, pulse (tachycardic, atrial fibrillation)	Palms (dry, rough, inelastic, cold, pale), pulse (bradycardic), carpal tunnel (positive Tinel's sign)
Eyes	Lid lag, lid retraction, exophthalmos/proptosis, ophthalmoplegia, chemosis	Periorbital puffiness, loss of outer one-third of eyebrows
Neck	Goitre, scars	Goitre, scars
Reflexes	Brisk	Delayed ankle jerks
Legs and skin	Pretibial myxoedema, vitiligo	

THYROID: EXAMINATION

On entering the room:

- Introduce yourself to the patient (permission)
- Obtain consent
- Obtain adequate exposure (position)
  - Position the chair well away from the wall so that you can get easily behind the patient to examine their neck.
  - Ask the patient to undo their top buttons to expose the upper chest so that you do not miss a midline sternotomy scar (from retrosternal goitre surgery) or distended/engorged veins on the chest wall (superior vena cava obstruction).
- Check if the patient has any pain (pain)
- Wash hands

Inspection

Look around the bed for clues, look at patient as a whole (thyroid status).

- Scars, tremor, myxoedema, wasting, periorbital puffiness, eye signs, swellings, asymmetry

Ask for a glass of water if there is not one visible.

Assess hoarseness of the voice by asking the patient to count from 1 to 10.

Ask them to take a deep breath in and listen for stridor.

Inspect the neck from the front, sides and back.

- Are there any obvious neck swellings or visible scars? Comment if the lump is in the anterior or posterior triangle.
- Ask the patient to open their mouth and stick out their tongue. If the swelling is a thyroglossal duct cyst, the upward tug when the patient protrudes their tongue is unmistakable. Note that the mouth must be open at the commencement of the test when the swelling is grasped. You may check for a lingual thyroid simultaneously at the base of the tongue whilst the patient's mouth is open.
- Ask the patient to take a sip of water, hold it in their mouth and swallow when you instruct them to, with their chin slightly elevated (Does the lump move with swallowing? If it does, it implies the swelling is thyroid-related).

Palpation from behind

Explain to the patient what you are about to do and then move behind them.

Ask again if it is tender.

Palpate from behind, but look at the patient's face when you start to press on the thyroid for signs of discomfort. Slightly flex the patient's head. Put one hand flat on one lobe and push it towards the midline. This will make the other side more prominent.

Check for the following:

- Tenderness
- Temperature
- Ask the patient to swallow again (this time ask yourself if you can you get below the thyroid gland when the patient swallows. If you can, it excludes retrosternal extension.)
- Size of goitre
- Consistency (soft, firm, hard; uniform or varied)
- Single, diffuse or multiple swellings
- Surface – Smooth or nodular (any prominent nodules?)
- Also check mobility and relation to surroundings (skin, trachea, muscle and carotid artery) for fixity, displacement and infiltration:
  - Gently pinch the skin over the thyroid to check for fixity
  - Check for fixation to the trachea (in two planes) and for tracheal displacement/ deviation
  - Check the relationship of the gland to the sternocleidomastoid muscle (ask the patient to look to one side and then gently push their chin down on the volar aspect of your wrist)
  - Assess the carotid artery pulsations (Berry's sign)

Examine regional lymph nodes

Submental, submandibular, deep cervical chain including the jugulodigastric group, supraclavicular, superficial cervical chain, pre-and post-auricular, occipital, pre-tracheal and pre-laryngeal groups.

Percussion

Percuss from the sternum upwards to check for retrosternal extension

Auscultation

Auscultate for a thyroid bruit (whilst the patient holds their breath)

Complete by:

- Assessing the patient's thyroid status and asking him or her some questions.
- Offering to check the patient's vocal cords by flexible laryngoscopy.
- Offering to perform Pemberton's test/sign – Ask the patient to elevate their arms above their head for 1 minute and look for congestion, cyanosis, stridor and distended neck veins, as a sign of a large retrosternal goitre.

Thank the patient and wash hands.

Summarise and offer your differential diagnosis.

THYROID GOITRES: DIFFERENTIAL DIAGNOSIS

Simple goitres:

- Physiological – Pregnancy, pubertal, lactation, menstruation
- Pathological – Iodine deficiency, goitrogens
- Multinodular goitre

Inflammatory:

- Thyroiditis (Hashimoto's, de Quervain's, Riedel's)

Neoplastic:

- Papillary
- Follicular/Hurthle
- Anaplastic
- Medullary
- Lymphoma

Toxic:

- Graves' goitre
- Solitary toxic adenoma/nodule
- Multinodular goitre (Plummer's disease)

Rare:

- TB, sarcoid, amyloid, HIV, lithium, amiodarone, syphilis

The solitary thyroid nodule

The differential diagnosis includes the following:

- Simple thyroid cyst
- Adenoma/simple hyperplastic nodule
- Prominent nodule in a multinodular goitre
- Enlarged lobe (e.g. Hashimoto's thyroiditis)
- Haemorrhage into a cyst/nodule
- Carcinoma – Primary or rarely secondary

PAROTID: EXAMINATION

Bear in mind that you may be asked to examine the neck and to pass the station you would be expected to pick up a lump in the tail of the parotid gland.

On entering the room:

- Introduce yourself to the patient (permission)
- Obtain consent
- Obtain adequate exposure (position)
- Check if the patient has any pain (pain)
- Wash hands

Inspection

Inspect both sides.

Look carefully for scars (the Blair incision is most often used so demonstrate to the examiners you are looking carefully in front of the tragus, in the preauricular skin crease and around the earlobe. If necessary, carefully lift up the earlobe).

Palpation

- Check if it is tender before proceeding.
- Define the characteristics of the lump, as you would for any other lump.

- Ask the patient to tense the underlying masseter muscle by getting them to clench their jaw and test for fixity.
- **Check the regional lymph node status** – If you suspect the lump is a preauricular lymph node, examine the face and scalp carefully for a primary site of infection or neoplasia.

Examine the oral cavity/oropharynx

Check for the following:

- The parotid duct (Stensen's duct) which lies opposite the upper second molar teeth (for pus, calculi etc.). Try to express pus out the parotid duct by gently massaging the gland and looking inside the oral cavity at the duct orifice.
- The oropharynx for evidence of medialisation of the tonsils from a deep parotid lobe tumour or a tumour sited in the parapharyngeal space.
- Offer to bimanually palpate the parotid gland (feeling the duct and the gland). However, its clinical value is limited compared with examination of the submandibular gland because the parotid lies behind the anterior edge of the masseter muscle and the vertical ramus of the mandible.

Check the integrity of the facial (VII) nerve

Ask the patient to 'raise their eyebrows', 'shut their eyes tight', 'blow out their cheeks', 'whistle', 'show you their teeth', 'grimace' and check taste sensation with respect to the anterior two-thirds of the tongue.

Complete by:

- Checking the contralateral side
- Testing sensation around the angle of the mandible and the earlobe if the patient has had a parotidectomy (great auricular nerve injury)
- Offering a full ENT examination

Differential diagnosis

Bear in mind that not every lump in the parotid region is a parotid gland swelling. When trying to formulate a differential diagnosis try to think what structures are in the immediate vicinity of the swelling, i.e.:

- Skin (sebaceous cyst, fungating squamous cell carcinoma)
- Subcutaneous tissue (lipoma, dermoid cyst)
- Muscle (masseter muscle hypertrophy)
- Facial nerve (neuroma)
- Lymphatics (preauricular lymph node)

- Bone (winging of mandible, prominent transverse process atlas/axis)
- Salivary tissue, i.e. tumours within the parotid gland itself (which may be benign or malignant)

Thank the patient and wash hands.

Summarise and offer your differential diagnosis.

In summary for a lesion in the parotid region, do not forget to

- Check the regional lymph node status
- Check the integrity of the facial nerve
- Look in the mouth

What are the complications of parotid surgery?

- Immediate – Permanent facial nerve injury (transaction), haematoma
- Early – Wound infection, flap necrosis, facial nerve weakness (temporary due to neuropraxia), salivary fistula, injury to the great auricular nerve
- Late – Wound dimple, Frey's syndrome (gustatory sweating due to misdirected reinnervation), recurrence

SUBMANDIBULAR SWELLING: EXAMINATION

On entering the room:

- Introduce yourself to the patient (permission)
- Obtain consent
- Obtain adequate exposure (position)
- Check if the patient has any pain (pain)
- Wash hands

Inspection

- Inspect both sides.
- Inspect carefully for scars and evidence of marginal mandibular nerve weakness.

Palpation

- Check if it is tender before proceeding.
- Define the characteristics of the lump, as you would for any other lump.
- To determine the relationship of the swelling to the mylohyoid muscle get the patient to tense the floor of the mouth (by asking the patient to push their tongue against the roof of their mouth). To determine the relationship to the sternocleidomastoid muscle, get the patient to contract this muscle.

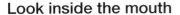

Look inside the mouth

- Check the submandibular (Wharton's) duct orifice under the tongue (for pus, calculi etc.).
- Look for evidence of dental infection or a primary carcinoma in the mouth (submental and submandibular lymph nodes drain the oral cavity).

Offer a bimanual palpation of the submandibular gland

- Before proceeding, ask for gloves. Generally, submandibular glands are ballottable whereas submandibular lymph nodes are not.
- Try to express pus out of the submandibular duct by gently massaging the gland and looking inside the oral cavity at the duct orifice.
- Test tongue sensation (lingual nerve) and mobility (hypoglossal nerve) – Malignant infiltration of nerves.
- Check regional lymph node status.
- Complete by

  - Checking the contralateral side and the parotid glands
  - Offering a full ENT examination

Thank the patient and wash hands.

Summarise and offer your differential diagnosis.

CHAPTER 7: LIMBS AND SPINE

MODEL FOR AN ORTHOPAEDIC HISTORY

Introduction

- Set the stage:
  - Welcome the patient. Ensure comfort and privacy.
  - Know and use the patient's name. Introduce and identify yourself.
- Set the agenda:
  - Begin with open-ended questions to ascertain the patient's perspective.
  - Encourage the consultations with silences and non-verbal and verbal cues.
  - Focus by paraphrasing and summarising.

Personal information

- Name, age, occupation, handedness and ethnic origin

Presenting complaint (in the patient's own words)

History of presenting complaint

- System specific:
  - Muscle, bone or joint pain (location, time, mode of onset, severity, nature, progression, quantity, quality, frequency, duration, relieving and exacerbating factors, associated symptoms, radiation)
  - Deformity
  - Swelling
  - Stiffness
  - Limb weakness
  - Reduced range of movement
  - Effects on function
- Risk factors
- Investigations and treatment
- Past medical, surgical and anaesthetic history
- Medication, allergies and immunisations
- Family history
- Social history
  - Marital status
  - Occupation and exposures
  - Smoking history
  - Alcohol consumption
  - Illicit drug use
  - Living accommodation
  - Recent travel history

System review

- General/constitutional
- Skin/breast
- Eyes/ears/nose/mouth/throat
- Cardiovascular
- Respiratory
- Gastrointestinal
- Genitourinary

- Musculoskeletal
- Neurological
- Psychiatrical
- Immunologic/lymphatic/endocrine

Thank the patient.

Summation

HIP JOINT: EXAMINATION

Introduction and handwash

- Start with the patient standing with a fully exposed hip joint.
- Ask the patient whether they have any pain.
- The examination of the hip (ball and socket) joint follows the same logical pattern as examination of any other joint. This includes

  - Look
  - Feel
  - Move
  - Special tests

Look

General

- Look around bed for walking aids and shoe-raises.
- Look at the patient as a whole. Well/unwell; pain/pain free.
- Assess gait. Note an Antalgic or Trendelenburg gait (see below).
- Assess posture – Assess for leg length inequality: True (due to a short leg) or apparent (result of a hip deformity) (see below).

Specific

- Inspect for swelling, muscle wasting, signs of inflammation and sinus formation.
- Anterior – Scars, wasting of quadriceps, sinuses, fixed flexion deformity (FFD) or rotational deformities. Put your hands on both anterior superior iliac spines (ASIS) to check if they are level (assess for pelvic tilt).
- Lateral – Scars, wasting muscles, sinuses and exaggerated lordosis of the spine.
- Posterior – Scars, wasting glutei/hamstrings, tufts of hair, scoliosis and sinuses.

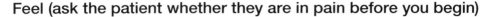

Feel (ask the patient whether they are in pain before you begin)

- Temperature of the joint (with the back of the hand).
- Palpate for local tenderness over this ball and socket joint and soft tissues.
- The hip joint lies posterior to the femoral artery at the mid-inguinal point (halfway between the ASIS and the symphysis pubis).
- Palpate the ischial tuberosity, greater trochanter and tendon of adductor longus
- Assess for inguinal lymph nodes.

Move (Figure 7.1)

- Assess for joint crepitus – Whilst moving the hip joint (with one hand over the hip joint, roll the femur laterally and medially).
- Perform *Thomas' test* (Figure 7.2).
- This test assesses for an FFD of the hip joint. Whilst the patient is in a supine position, place your hand between the patient's lumbar supine and the examination couch. Obliterate the lumbar lordosis by flexing the patient's good hip (ask the patient to bring their knee up towards their chest and hold it). This should compress your hand between their lumbar spine and the couch. The opposite leg should remain flat on the couch. Now you may exclude an FFD of the bad hip. The opposite leg will lift off the couch demonstrating the amount of flexion deformity present.
- Hip flexion has already been assessed in Thomas' test. The normal range of hip flexion is 0°–120°.
- Test for abduction/adduction of the hip, whilst immobilising the pelvis by placing your hand on the contralateral ASIS to fix the pelvis. Then abduct (45°) and adduct (25°) each hip. Assess the range of movement and note any crepitus.
- Test for internal and external rotation (in extension) by looking at the patellae (90° arc of movement). Assess the range of movement and note any crepitus.
- Test internal (30°) and external (45°) rotation with the hip flexed (flex the hip and knee to 90°). Assess the range of movement and note any crepitus.

Special tests

Trendelenburg's test (Figure 7.3)

Face the standing patient. Have the patient rest their hands on your shoulders. This will support the patient and prevent them from falling over. Put your hands on their ASIS to assess for a pelvic tilt. First, ask the patient to stand on their good leg whilst flexing the non-weight-bearing leg at the knee to 90°. Then repeat the test on the other leg. When a person stands on one leg, the glutei muscles contract so the opposite side of the pelvis is titled up slightly to allow the leg to clear the ground on walking.

Positive Trendelenburg sign: If the actions of the glutei muscles are deficient, the opposite side of the pelvis will tilt downwards and the patient maintains balances by leaning over towards the side of the problem.

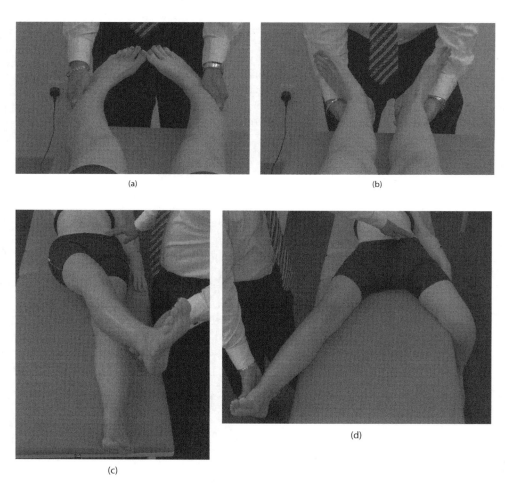

Figure 7.1 Hip movements: (a) internal rotation; (b) external rotation; (c) adduction; (d) abduction.

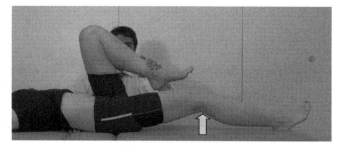

Figure 7.2 Modified Thomas' test for assessing a fixed flexion deformity. A fixed flexion deformity of the right hip is indicated by an inability to fully straighten the right leg (arrow).

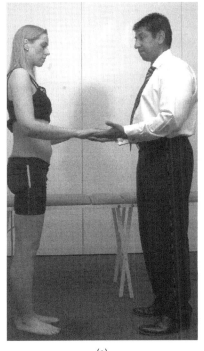
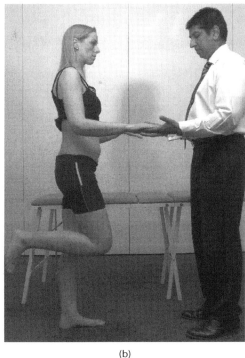

(a)   (b)

Figure 7.3 (a) and (b) Trendelenburg test.

Assess leg lengths

The patient should be in a supine position. Square the pelvis and place legs in comparable positions. A fixed flexion deformity of the hip joint is present when the legs are unequal in length when they are in a parallel position.

Apparent leg length is measured between fixed points, for example from the xiphisternum or umbilicus to the tip of the malleolus.

True leg length is measured from the ASIS to the medial malleolus.

The *Galleazi test* is performed with the patient's heels together. Examine the patient from the side and the end of the examination couch. Assess if the leg shortening originates from the femur (above knee) or the tibia (below knee). If you are unclear, flex the hip and knee joints to 90° and look at the knees from the side.

Complete the hip joint examination

- Assess the neurovascular status of the lower limbs.
- Examine the joint above and below (spine/knee).

- Assess the impact of the joint condition on the patient's life.
- Request an x-ray of the hip joint.
- Assess the patient's fitness for surgery.

Thank the patient and wash hands.

Summarise and offer your differential diagnosis.

KNEE JOINT: EXAMINATION

Introduction and handwash

Start with the patient standing and fully expose the knee joint.

Ask the patient whether they have any pain.

The examination of the knee (hinge) joint follows the same logical pattern as examination of any other joint. This includes

- Look
- Feel
- Move
- Special tests

Look

General

- Look around bed for walking aids, shoe-raises etc.
- Look at the patient as a whole (well/unwell; pain/pain free).
- Ask the patient to walk and squat.

Specific

Whilst the patient is standing:

- Inspect for swelling, muscle wasting, signs of inflammation and sinus formation.
- Anterior with the legs together – Scars, wasting of quadriceps muscle, sinuses, FFD/deformities and valgus/varus deformities (alignment).
- Lateral – Scars, wasting muscles, sinuses and FFD.
- Posterior – Scars and popliteal swellings.

Whilst the patient is supine:

- Inspect for effusion – Look for a 'horseshoe' swelling of the suprapatellar pouch.
- Inspect for scars, including arthroscopic scars either side of the patella tendon, anteromedially and anterolaterally.

Feel (ask the patient whether they are in pain before you begin)

- Temperature of the joint (with the back of your hand).
- If you noted quadriceps muscle wasting on inspection, now measure the leg circumference 15 cm above the tibial tubercle.
- Ask the patient to push their heels down into the bed and feel the bulk of the quadriceps muscle. To exclude an FFD, place your hand behind the popliteal fossa. If an FFD is present, place one hand on patella and one hand on quadriceps muscle and straighten the knee joint to confirm it is fixed.
- Assess for a knee joint effusion

    For small effusions, perform the *'swipe test'* and inspect for loss of the medial sulcus. For moderate effusions, perform the *'patellar tap test'*. With the knee extended, empty the suprapatellar pouch by pressure of your hand. With your other hand, press against the patella sharply against the femur to produce a 'tap'.
    For large effusions, ballot the fluid between the medial and lateral aspects of the joint ('*cross fluctuation test*').

- Palpate for local tenderness over this hinge joint and soft tissues

    Flex the patient's knee to 45° and palpate this joint systematically (medial tibial condyle, medial joint line, medial femoral condyle, medial collateral ligament, tibial tuberosity, posteriorly in the popliteal fossa, lateral femoral condyle, lateral joint line, lateral tibial condyle, lateral collateral ligament and head of the fibula). Now straighten the knee joint and palpate the patella in two planes (assess for patellofemoral joint crepitus and tenderness).

- Palpate along the extensor mechanism for gaps or defects.
- Assess for popliteal lymph nodes.

Move

- Place your hand on the knee joint to detect crepitus on movement and then ask the patient to flex the knee (bring the patient's heel to their bottom). The range of movement is 0°–150°. At the limit of movement, assess the range of passive movement (Figure 7.4).
- Inspect for an intact extension apparatus, flexion contractures and 'extensor lag' on straight leg raising. Ask the patient to point their toes to the ceiling, perform a straight leg raise and then return the leg to the examination couch.
- Assess for hyperextension (genu recurvatum) by placing your hand on the patient's patella and lift their heel upwards.

Special Tests

- Collateral ligaments (Figure 7.5)

    - *Valgus/varus stress* – With the patient's knee fully extended, hold the patient's ankle in your axilla. With both of your hands, abduct and adduct the femur whilst keeping the patient's knee joint in extension and then in flexion.

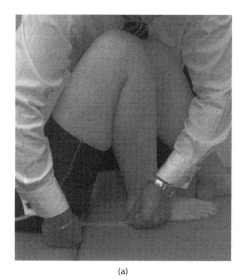

(a)

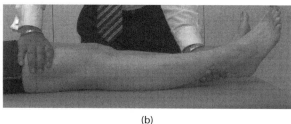

(b)

Figure 7.4 (a) Knee flexion and (b) extension.

- Cruciate ligaments
  - *Posterior sag test* – Place the patient's heels together, knees flexed to 45° and inspect from the side.
  - *Drawer test* – With the patient's knees flexed to 45°, inform and then sit on the patient's feet (Figure 7.7).
    Excessive anterior draw is due to laxity of the anterior cruciate and posterior lag is associated with laxity of the posterior cruciate ligament.
  - *Lachman's test* – Flex the patient's knee to 20°. Hold the lower end of the thigh in your one hand and the upper end of the tibia with the other. Push the lower thigh in one direction and pull the tibia in the opposite direction and then in the reverse directions (Figure 7.6).
- Menisci
  - *McMurray's test* – Flex and externally rotate the knee and then slowly extend the knee to stress the medial meniscus. Flex and internally rotate the knee and then slowly extend the knee to stress the lateral meniscus. Palpate for click and assess for focal tenderness during the test as it may suggest a tear.

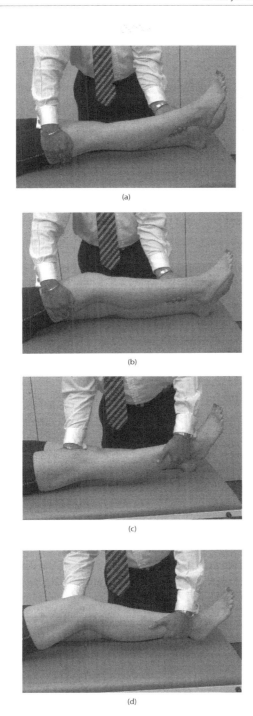

Figure 7.5 Assessing the medial (a) and (b) and lateral (c, d) collateral ligaments.

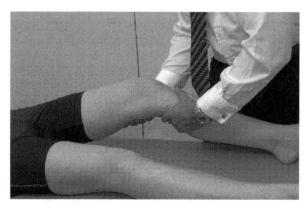

Figure 7.6 Lachmann's test: flex the knee to 15°–30° and pull the proximal tibia forwards.

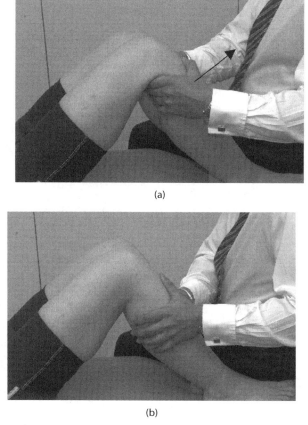

(a)

(b)

Figure 7.7 (a) Anterior draw test for anterior cruciate ligament stability; (b) posterior draw test for posterior cruciate ligament stability.

- Patella
  - *Lateral apprehension test* – With the patient's knee in extension, apply pressure against the medial border of the patella. Maintain the pressure, whilst flexing the knee to 30°and assess the degree of patella movement. Inspect the patient's face for apprehension.

Complete the knee joint examination

- Assess the neurovascular status of the lower limbs.
- Examine the joint above and below (spine/hip/ankle joints).
- Assess the impact of the joint condition on the patient's life.
- Request a weight-bearing x-ray of the knee joint.
- Assess the patient's fitness for surgery.

Thank the patient and wash hands.

Summarise and offer your differential diagnosis.

SHOULDER JOINT: EXAMINATION

Introduction and handwash

Start with the patient standing and fully expose the shoulder joint.

Ask the patient whether they have any pain.

The examination of the shoulder (ball and socket) joint follows the same logical pattern as examination of any other joint. This includes

- Look
- Feel
- Move
- Special tests

Look

General

- Look around bed for aids (slings).
- Look at the patient as a whole (well/unwell; pain/pain free).

Specific

Whilst the patient is standing:

- Inspect for swelling, muscle wasting, signs of inflammation and sinus formation.
- Anterior – Arthroscopic scars, sinuses, contour of the shoulder/squaring off, muscle wasting of deltoid and trapezius.

- Lateral – Scars.
- Posterior – Scars, contour and muscle wasting of supraspinatus/ infraspinatus.
- Ask the patient to push with their hands against a wall. Inspect for winging of the scapula (serratus anterior muscle supplied by long thoracic nerve of Bell, C5/6/7).

Feel (ask the patient whether they are in pain before you begin)

- Temperature of the joint (with the back of the hand).
- Palpate over the sternoclavicular joint (SCJ), along the clavicle, coracoid process, acromion/acromioclavicular joint (ACJ), subacromial space, abduct the humerus and then palpate the glenohumeral joint line into the axilla. Continue posteriorly to assess the greater tuberosity of humerus, spine of scapula, inferior pole of scapula, supraspinatus and infraspinatus.
- Assess for axillary lymph nodes.

Move (Figure 7.9)

- Place your hand on the shoulder joint to detect crepitus on passive movement and then ask the patient to flex the knee (bring the patient's heel to their bottom). The range of movement is 0°–150°. At the limit of movement, assess the range of passive movement.
- Forward flexion. With the patient's arm by the side, ask the patient to flex the shoulder forward (90°).
- Abduction. Ask the patient to abduct the arm (90°). Assess for a 'painful arc'.
- Adduction. Ask the patient to bring their arm over to the opposite shoulder (assess for osteoarthritis [OA] of ACJ at this point = *Scarf test*).
- Extension.
- External rotation. Flex the patient's elbows to 90° and then ask the patient to place their hands behind their head.
- Internal rotation. Ask the patient to place their hands behind their back (normally one should be able to reach up as high as the sixth thoracic vertebrae).

Special tests

- *Rotator cuff* muscles

  - *Supraspinatus* (thumbs down test/Jobe's test/Empty can test). Ask the patient to abduct their arm against resistance (Figure 7.10). To exclude rupture, passively abduct the patient's arm to 40°, then the patient should be able to continue active abduction.
  - *Teres minor* and *infraspinatus*-resisted external rotation.
  - *Subscapularis* – Gerber's lift-off test.

- *Impingement test* – This is impairment of rotator cuff function within the subacromial bursa. It may lead to inflammation or a partial or full thickness tear. Impingement is characterised by pain and weakness on abduction and internal rotation.
    - *Neer's sign and test* – With the patient's thumb down, place your hand on their shoulder and with your other hand passively lift up their hand in the plane of the scapula (forward flexion) until they express pain (Figure 7.12b). Pain during this manoeuvre is a positive *Neer's sign* and pain abolished with local anaesthetic is a positive *Neer's test*.
    - *Hawkin's test* – Raise the patient's arm to 90° forward flexion and bend the elbow to 90°. Then passively internally rotate the shoulder (i.e. thumb pointed down) (Figure 7.12a). Pain is indicative of impingement.
    - *Jobe's test (empty can)* – Ask the patient to abduct the arc to 90° elevation in the scapula plane with full internal rotation (empty can). Ask the patient to resist downward pressure. The presence of pain is a positive test.
- *Ruptured head of biceps*
    - Assess for a 'biceps bulge' on flexing the patient's elbow against resistance.
- *Axillary nerve function*
    - Assess for deltoid muscle power and sensation (fine touch) in regimental badge area (Figure 7.8).

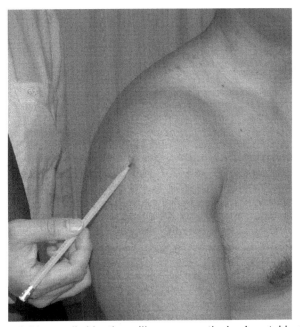

Figure 7.8 The area of skin supplied by the axillary nerve – the 'regimental badge area'.

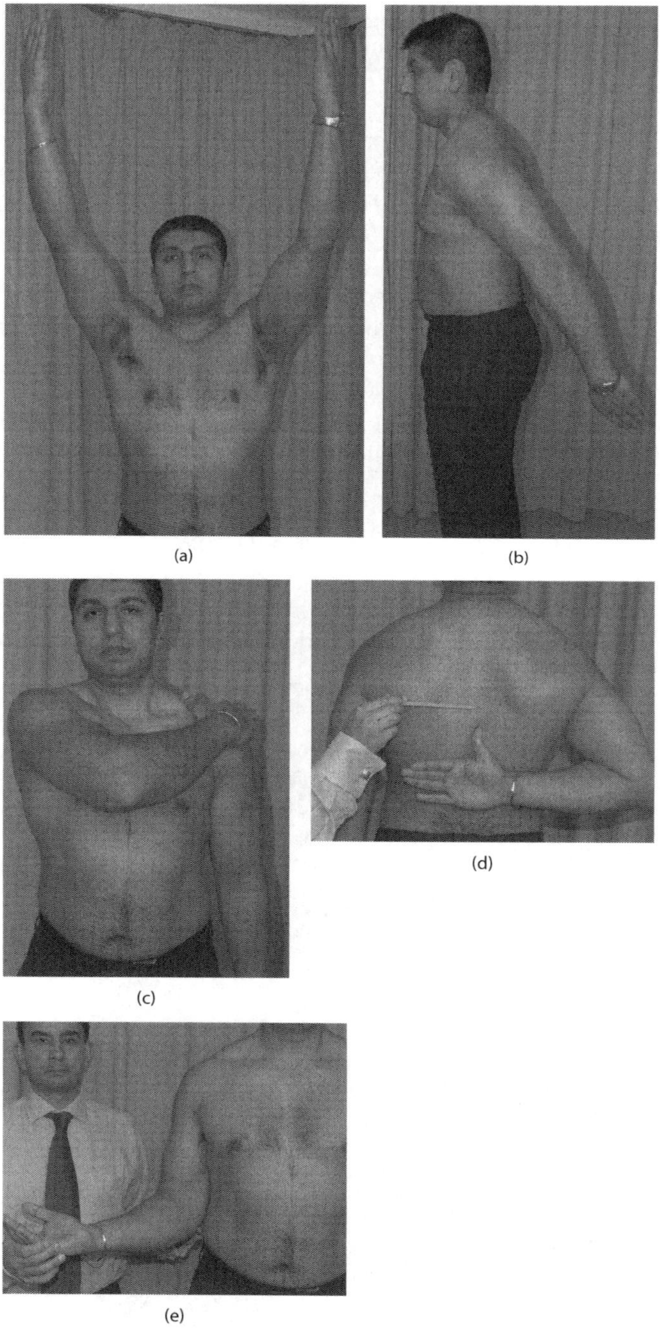

Figure 7.9 Movements of the shoulder: (a) forward flexion; (b) extension; (c) adduction; (d) internal rotation; (e) external rotation.

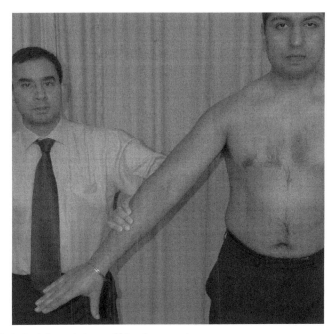

Figure 7.10 Jobe's test for rotator cuff impingement.

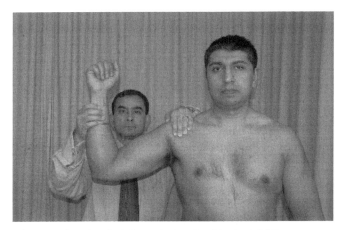

Figure 7.11 Anterior apprehension test for anterior shoulder instability.

Complete the shoulder joint examination

- Offer to perform apprehension test to test for shoulder instability (Figure 7.11).
- Assess the neurovascular status of the upper limbs.
- Examine the joint above and below (cervical spine and elbow joint).

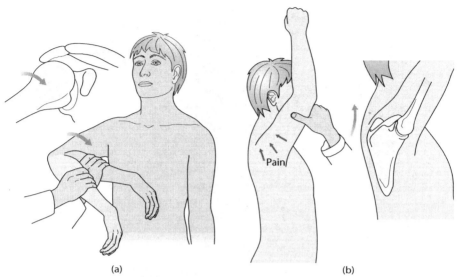

(a)   (b)

Figure 7.12 (a) Hawkin's impingement test. Impingement pain is reproduced when the shoulder is internally rotated with 90° of forward flexion, thereby locating the greater tuberosity underneath the acromion; (b) Neer's impingement test. Pain is reproduced with full forward flexion.

- Assess the impact of the joint condition on the patient's life.
- Request x-rays (including axillary view) of the shoulder joint.
- Assess the patient's fitness for surgery.

Thank the patient and wash hands.

Summarise and offer your differential diagnosis.

HANDS: EXAMINATION

Introduction and handwash

Start with the patient sitting. The patient's upper limbs should be fully exposed and their hands resting on a pillow.

Ask the patient whether they have any pain.

The hand examination may represent a rheumatologic, orthopaedic, neurological or vascular case. In this section, we focus on the 'Rheumatoid hand' examination.

The examination of the hands follows the same logical pattern as examination of any other joint. This includes

- Look
- Feel
- Move
- Special tests

Look

General

- Look around bed for aids and supports.
- Look at the patient as a whole (well/unwell; pain/pain free).
- Ensure you assess for extra-articular manifestations of systemic disease (see below).

Specific

Dorsal aspect of the patient's hands

- Skin and soft tissue
  - Nail changes (nail fold infarcts, pitting, vasculitic lesions, pale beds)
  - Ulcers
  - Rashes
  - Bruising, purpura and thinning of the skin (secondary to steroids)
  - Swelling
- Muscles
  - Wasting of intrinsic muscles (accentuates the extensor tendons)
  - Dorsal guttering
- Bones
  - Loss of the normal finger cascade
  - Spindling of fingers
  - Sparing of distal interphalangeal (DIP) joints
  - Ulnar deviation of fingers (Figure 7.15)
  - Swan-neck deformity (hyperextended proximal interphalangeal [PIP] joint but flexed DIP joint)
  - Boutonniere deformity (flexed PIP joint, extended metacarpophalangeal [MCP] joint, hyperextended DIP joint)
  - MCP joints and wrist subluxation
  - Radial deviation and volar subluxation at the wrist joint
  - Z-deformities of the thumbs
  - Heberden's (DIP joints) and Bouchard's nodes (PIP joints) and squaring off of the thumb indicating OA (Figure 7.16)

Palmar/volar aspect of the patient's hands

Ask the patient to lift their hands off the pillow in order to expose the palmar aspects of their hands. Assess for a dropped finger/thumb (evidence of extensor tendon rupture) and wrist drop. Moreover, assess for range of movement (supination/pronation).

- Skin and deep fascia
  - Scars (carpal tunnel decompression; a dorsal wrist scar implies previous synovectomy or arthrodesis in rheumatoid arthritis [RA]; a scar over the head of the ulna implies a previous Darrach procedure)
  - Pale palmar creases
  - Palmar erythema
- Muscles
  - Wasting of the thenar and hypothenar eminences (Figure 7.14)
- Bones
  - Fingers held in flexion
- Elbows

- *Ask the patient to put their hands behind their head and check for*

  - Scars around the medial epicondyle (ulnar nerve decompression)
  - Rheumatoid nodules

Feel (ask the patient whether they are in pain before you begin)

- Temperature of the hands (with the back of the hand).
- Capillary refill time and assess ulnar and radial pulses.
- Squeeze the metacarpals together and assess for tenderness.
- Palpate each joint to ascertain the levels affected in the hand and whether active inflammation or inactive disease is present.
- Palpate for rheumatoid nodules (i.e. on pressure areas and tendon sheaths).
- Palpate for tendon ruptures (start your palpation on the ulnar side of the hands).

Move

Assess for active and passive movement at the wrist and fingers.

Ask the patient to perform the following movements:

- Grip and squeeze two of your fingers and perform a fine pinch.
- Flex one finger at a time whilst touching the thenar eminence.
- Spread their fingers wide apart.
- Demonstrate playing the piano with their fingers.
- Oppose thumb to each finger.
- Place their hands in a 'pray position' to demonstrate wrist dorsiflexion (Figure 7.13a).
- Place their hands in a 'reverse pray position' to demonstrate wrist flexion (Figure 7.13b).

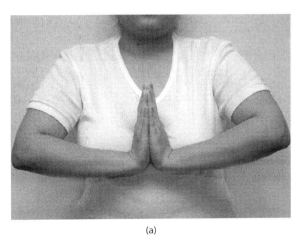

(a)

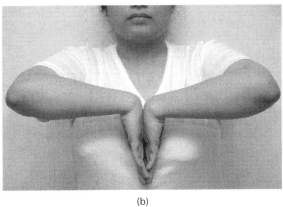

(b)

Figure 7.13 Testing the range of (a) wrist extension and (b) wrist flexion.

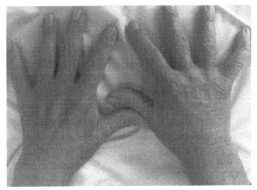

Figure 7.14 Intrinsic muscle wasting due to ulnar neuropathy.

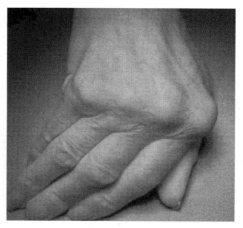

Figure 7.15 Rheumatoid hand showing ulnar drift at the metacarpophalangeal joints.

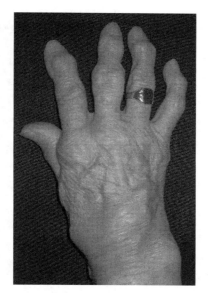

Figure 7.16 Hand deformities secondary to osteoarthritis.

Special tests

Functional assessment:

- Power grip
- Pincer grip (pick up a coin or key)
- Button and unbutton shirt
- Hold a pen and write

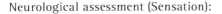

Neurological assessment (Sensation):

- Radial nerve (dorsum of first interosseous webspace)
- Median nerve (palmar/volar aspect of index finger)
- Ulnar nerves (palmar/volar aspect of little finger)

Table top test:

- Ask the patient to place their hands flat on a table.

Extra-articular manifestations of rheumatoid disease:

- Systemic – Weight loss, fever, malaise, vasculitis and amyloidosis
- Skin – Subcutaneous (rheumatoid) nodules
- Eyes – Keratoconjunctivitis sicca, scleritis, episcleritis
- Cardiovascular – Pericardial effusion, pericarditis, myocarditis
- Respiratory – Pleurisy, pleural effusion, nodules and fibrosing alveolitis
- Neurological – Entrapment neuropathy (carpal tunnel syndrome), atlantoaxial instability and multifocal neuropathies
- Abdominal – Splenomegaly, Felty's syndrome
- Haematological – Anaemia, leucopenia and lymphadenopathy
- Muscular-Skeletal – Knees (valgus/varus deformity, popliteal 'Baker's' cysts), scars for shoulder, knee or hip replacements

Complete the hand examination

- Perform a full neurological assessment of the upper limbs.
- Perform a full vascular examination of the upper limbs.
- Examine the joint above (wrist and elbow joints).
- Assess other joint involvement (hip, knee, shoulder, spine).
- Assess for extra-articular manifestations of rheumatoid disease (eyes, respiratory, cardiovascular, neurological systems).
- Assess the impact of the joint condition on the patient's life.
- Request x-rays of wrist and hand.
- Assess the patient's fitness for surgery.

Thank the patient and wash hands.

Summarise and offer your differential diagnosis.

SPINE: EXAMINATION

Introduction and handwash

Start with the patient standing and fully exposed.

Ask the patient whether they have any pain.

The examination of the spine follows the same logical pattern as examination of any other joint. This includes

- Look
- Feel
- Move
- Special tests

Look

General

- Look around bed for walking aids and supports (Miami J collar, thoracolumbar brace).
- Look at the patient as a whole (well/unwell; pain/pain free).
- Ask the patient to walk in order to assess gait.
- Ask the patient to stand on their heels (L4–L5) and toes (S1–S2).

Specific

Whilst the patient is standing, inspect

- Skin – Scars, sinuses, hairy tufts, café au lait spots
- Soft tissues – Muscle wasting
- Bone – Scoliosis, kyphosis, lumbar lordosis, gibbus

Feel

- Ask the patient whether they are in pain before you begin.
- Temperature of the spine (with the back of the hand).
- Palpate and percuss over the entire spine for any bony or muscle tenderness and assess for step deformities.

Move

Cervical spine (Figure 7.17):

- Ask the patient to move the head forward and backward (flexion 75° and extension 60°).
- Ask the patient to look to the right and left (80° each direction).
- Ask the patient to tilt their head to the right and left towards their ear (lateral flexion 45° each direction).

Thoracic spine:

- Ask the patient to rotate whilst sitting.
- Measure chest expansion.

Lumbar spine (Figure 7.19):

- *Forward flexion* – Ask the patient to touch their toes (if reduced, perform *Schober's test*). The patient should be able to reach within 7 cm of the floor.
- *Extension* – Ask the patient to bend backward (30°).

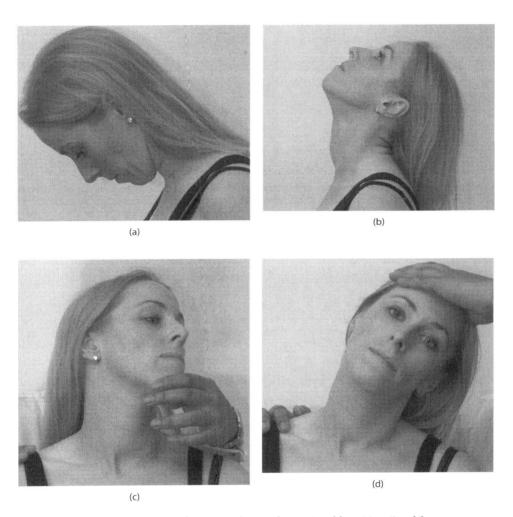

Figure 7.17 Cervical spine flexion/extension (a and b), rotation (c) and bending (d).

- *Lateral flexion* – Ask the patient to slide their hand down one side of the body (30°).
- *Rotation* – Ask the patient to sit down, cross their hands across their body and rotate their body (40°).

Special tests

Cervical spine

- *Lhermitte's sign (the barber-chair phenomenon)* is demonstrated when you ask the patient to bend their cervical neck forward. This produces a radicular pain down the spine and into the upper limb. A positive test represents cervical nerve root compression.

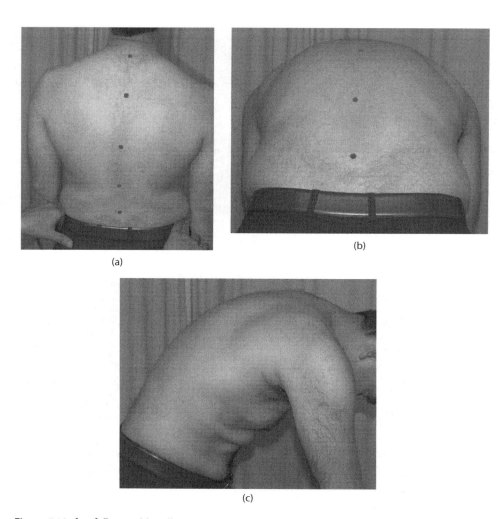

(a)

(b)

(c)

Figure 7.18 (a–c) Forward bending test.

- *Spurling's test* is used to demonstrate cervical nerve root entrapment. Extend the cervical spine and rotate the head to each shoulder in turn. The presence of a shooting pain down the arm may indicate cervical root compression.

Lumbar spine

- *Straight leg raise and sciatic nerve test (Lasègue's straight leg test; Figure 7.20):* Examine patient in a supine position. With the patient's knee flexed, first check passive hip flexion is normal. With the patient's knees extended, raise the patient's leg whilst supporting the patient's heel. On the affected side, the patient will

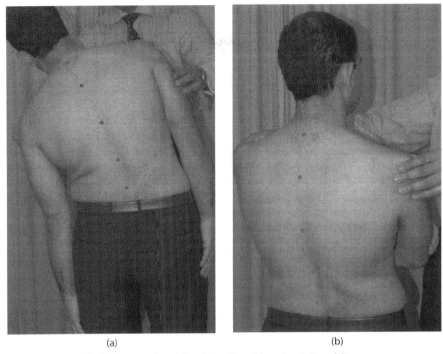

(a)   (b)

Figure 7.19 Lumbar flexion/extension, lateral bending (a) and rotation (b).

experience pain at a certain level. At this limit, gently dorsiflex the ankle, which will apply further tension on the nerve root (Bragard's sign). Ensure you measure the angle the leg is elevated off the examination couch.

- *Femoral stretch test* – Ask the patient to lie prone. Flex the patient's knee and ask the patient to inform you when they have pain. The test is positive if the patient has pain radiating into their back.
- *Modified Schober's test (Figure 7.18)* (mark the level between the iliac crests and 10 cm above, ask the patient to touch their toes. There should be >5 cm increase in separation).
- *Heel-hips-occiput test* also known as the 'wall test' (ankylosing spondylitis [AS]).
- *Patrick's test* for sacro-iliac joint (SIJ) (also known as the *Faber test*) and other SIJ tests.

Complete the spine examination

- Perform a full neurological assessment of the upper and lower limbs.
- Perform a full vascular examination of the upper and lower limbs.
- Perform an abdominal examination (to exclude an abdominal aortic aneurysm) and assess anal tone by performing a digital rectal examination.

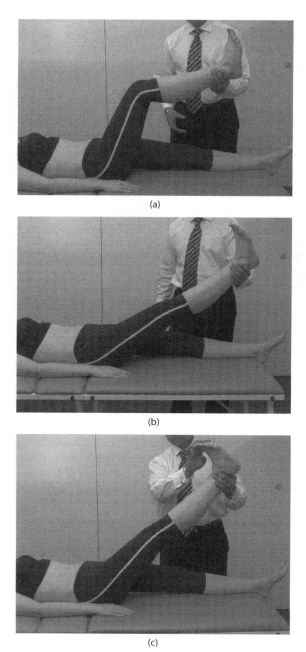

(a)

(b)

(c)

Figure 7.20 (a–c) Lasègue's straight leg test.

- Examine the joint above and below (shoulder and hip joint).
- Assess the impact of the joint condition on the patient's life.
- Request x-rays of the spine. Further imaging, including computed tomography (CT) and magnetic resonance imaging (MRI) scans should be considered.
- Assess the patient's fitness for surgery.

Thank the patient and wash hands.

Summarise and offer your differential diagnosis.

CHAPTER 8:
NEUROSCIENCES

MODEL FOR A NEUROLOGICAL HISTORY

Introduction

- Set the stage
  - Welcome the patient. Ensure comfort and privacy.
  - Know and use the patient's name. Introduce and identify yourself.

- Set the agenda
  - Begin with open-ended questions to ascertain the patient's perspective.
  - Encourage the consultations with silences and non-verbal and verbal cues.
  - Focus by paraphrasing and summarizing.
- Set the objective – Obtain the diagnosis
  1. Physiological diagnosis *(What is the lesion?)*
     - Cortical
     - Spinal cord
     - Peripheral nervous system (PNS) (upper motor neuron [UMN]/lower motor neuron [LMN], motor/sensory, diffuse/focal)
  2. Anatomical diagnosis (*Where is the lesion?*)
  3. Pathological diagnosis

Personal information

- Name, age, gender, handedness, occupation and ethnic origin.

Presenting complaint (in the patient's own words)

History of presenting complaint

- Chronological order of the symptoms – Time course, onset, duration, frequency, progression, location, quality, quantity, severity, aggravating and relieving factors and associated symptoms.
- System specific
  - Motor changes – Weakness, clumsiness, stiffness, paralysis, tremor and disturbances in gait
  - Sensory changes – Numbness, paraesthesia and temperature changes
  - Pain – Location, time, mode of onset, severity, nature, progression, quantity, quality, frequency, duration, relieving and exacerbating factors, associated symptoms and radiation
  - Headache
  - Nausea or vomiting
  - Loss or altered consciousness
  - Seizures
  - Visual disturbances
  - Behavioural changes
- Risk factors for the presenting complaint
- Investigations and treatment provided to date

Past medical, surgical and anaesthetic history

Use the mnemonic: THREADS MIJ

- Tuberculosis
- Hypertension
- Rheumatic fever/Rheumatoid arthritis
- Epilepsy
- Asthma
- Diabetes
- Stroke
- Myocardial Infarction
- Jaundice

Medication, allergies and immunisations

Family history

First-degree relatives with relevant familial diseases – Muscular dystrophy, spinocerebellar degeneration, Huntington's chorea and diabetes mellitus.

Social history

- Marital status
- Occupation and exposures
- Smoking history (number of pack-years)
- Alcohol intake (units/week)
- Recreational drug use
- Living accommodation
- Level of support (family and carers)
- Recent travel history

System review

During your targeted history taking, ask only the relevant questions based on the patient's history.

- General/constitutional
- Skin/breast
- Eyes/ears/nose/mouth/throat
- Cardiovascular
- Respiratory
- Gastrointestinal
- Genitourinary
- Musculoskeletal

- Psychiatrical
- Immunologic/lymphatic/endocrine

Thank the patient.

Summation

THE CRANIAL NERVE EXAMINATION

Introduction and handwash

- Have the patient sitting up in the examination couch or chair.
- Ask the patient whether they have any pain. Take note of their speech.

Inspection

General

- Look around bed for aids (walking, hearing).
- Look at the patient as a whole (well/unwell; pain/pain free).

Specific

- Inspection for involuntary movements (tremor, fasciculation, choreiform).
- Inspect facial appearances (weakness, asymmetrical, ptosis).
- Listen for dysphasia (expressive, receptive).

Olfactory (I) Nerve:

- Test the sense of smell. Apply peppermint, vanilla and coffee to each nostril.

Optic (II) Nerve:

- Test visual acuity using the Snellen chart. Test each eye separately.
- Test pupillary reflexes by examining the pupils in a darkened room. Assess for size, symmetry. Assess direct and consensual reflex in each eye in turn with the use of a pen torch. Test accommodation by asking the patient to look into the distance and then focus on an object close to their face. Test for changes in pupil size.
- Test visual fields by confrontation. You may use a red hat pin to perform this test.
- Perform fundoscopy in a dark room using an ophthalmoscope. Demonstrate the 'red reflex' by shining the light in each pupil and then examine each fundi, optic discs and macula.

Oculomotor (III), Trochlear (IV) and Abducent (VI) Nerves

- Test each eye for ocular movements whilst holding the patient's head in a neutral position.
- Assess for strabismus or nystagmus (vertical, horizontal or rotatory).
- Ask the patient to follow your finger up and down, right (up and down) and then left (up and down). Then assess the six points in an 'H' pattern.
- Ask the patient to report diplopia. If present, ask the patient to close each eye in turn to identify the side of the false image.
- Assess convergence by asking the patient to focus on your finer as it is brought in from a distance towards the tip of their nose.

Trigeminal (V) nerve

Motor function:

- Test the muscles of mastication for wasting.
- Assess jaw strength (ask the patient to open their jaw against resistance).
- Palpate masseters for bulk and symmetry.

Sensory function:

- Assess sensation (fine touch, temperature) in the three divisions (ophthalmic, maxillary, mandibular) and compare both sides of the face.
- Test the corneal reflex with a cotton wool tip.

Jaw jerk:

- Place your finger in the midline over the tip of the patient's mandible, with the patient's mouth slightly open. Tap over finger with a tendon hammer.

Facial (VII) nerve

- Assess for facial asymmetry and spontaneous movements (spasm).
- Inspect for symmetry of eye blinking and closure.

Motor function:

- Assess the facial muscles. Ask the patient to raise their eyebrows, wrinkle forehead (frown), close their eyes, smile, show their teeth, blow out their cheeks and pucker their lips.

Sensory function (taste):

- Test the anterior two-thirds of each side of the patient's tongue (using sweet/salt, bitter/or sour). This tests the chorda tympani nerve.

Schirmer's test:

- Test tear secretion. Place a piece of tissue paper under the lower eyelid and remove after 5 minutes.

Vestibulocochlear (VIII) nerve

Hearing function:

- Test hearing in both ears by asking the patient to repeat a whispered word.
- Perform Rinne's test (air vs. bone conduction) in each ear by placing vibrating tuning forks on mastoid process and lateral to external ear. Ask the patient which sound is louder.
- Perform Weber's test (lateralizing sign) in each ear by placing a vibrating turning fork over the middle of the patient's forehead. Ask the patient where the sound is loudest (midline or to the side).
- Examine the ear with an auroscope (external acoustic canal, tympanic membranes).

Vestibular function:

- Perform the oculocephalic reflex ('doll's eye'). Ensure no wax is present in the ear canal. Irrigate saline (30° or 44°) into the canal and observe for an eye response. A normal response to cold water irrigation is for the patient to develop nystagmus towards the contralateral side. A normal response to warm water irrigation is for the patient to develop nystagmus towards the ipsilateral side.

Glossopharyngeal (IX) and vagus (X) nerves

- Assess palate and uvula function by asking the patient to say 'Aah'.
- Assess tactile sensation of the tonsil, palate and upper pharynx with a tongue depressor.
- Perform gag reflex on each side.
- Assess the patient's voice (volume, quality) and phonation.
- Ask the patient to cough and swallow.

Spinal accessory (XI) nerve

- Inspect the trapezius muscle for tone and bulk. Ask the patient to shrug their shoulders and repeat against resistance.
- Inspect sternomastoid for tone and bulk. Ask the patient to turn their head and repeat against resistance.

Hypoglossal (XII) nerve

- Ask the patient to protrude their tongue. Assess for symmetry, bulk, wasting or fasciculations. The tongue will deviate to the affected side.
- Assess strength on lateral deviation by asking the patient to move their tongue from side to side and then assess bulk and contraction strength.

Thank the patient and wash hands

Summarise and offer your differential diagnosis

Summary of cranial nerve (I-XII) examination

I Olfactory

Assess the patient's sense of smell by testing each nostril in turn. Essence bottles of coffee, vanilla and peppermint.

II Optic

- General – Observe for pupil asymmetry, ptosis and swelling.
- Visual acuity – If the patient wears glasses, keep them on. Test each eye separately using a Snellen chart.
- Visual fields – Stand 2 feet in front of the patient and ensure you are at eye level. Move your hands to side half way between yourself and the patient, wiggle fingers, ask the patient when they see movement. Assess nasal and temporal fields.
- Fundoscopy – Assess the funds, macula and optic discs.

III, IV VI Oculomotor, Trochlear, Abducens

- Inspect the pupils – Shape, size and ptosis.
- Pupil reaction – To light reaction (direct, consensual and swinging light test) and accommodation.
- Extra-ocular eye movements – Assess saccadic and pursuit movements.

V Trigeminal

- Facial sensation – On forehead, cheek and jaw
- Motor – Check for the following muscles: Temporalis, masseter and pterygoids
- Ask the patient to open their mouth and clench their teeth
- Bite strength
- Corneal reflex
- Jaw jerk

VII Facial

- Inspect for a facial droop or asymmetry.
- Facial expression – Ask the patient to look up and wrinkle their forehead. Inspect for wrinkling loss. Ask the patient to shut their eyes tightly. Ask the patient to smile and look for asymmetry in their nasolabial folds. In addition, ask the patient to frown, show their teeth and puff out their cheeks. Assess for taste.

VIII Vestibulocochlear

- Auditory acuity of each ear – Place your hands by each ear of the patient. Rub your fingers to create noise on one side and keep the other hand still, then switch hands. Ask the patient, which ear they hear the noise. If hearing loss is identified, inspect the external auditory canals and the tympanic membranes.

Rinne's test (air vs. bone conduction)

- Apply tuning fork (512 Hz) on the mastoid behind ear. Ask the patient when they can no longer hear the sound. Then move the tuning fork neck to the patient's ear canal so they can hear the sound. A normal response is that air conduction (ear) is better heard than bone conduction (mastoid).

Weber's test (lateralization)
Apply tuning fork (256 Hz) to the top of patient's head on middle of forehead. Ask the patient 'where do you hear the sound coming from?' A normal response is in the midline.

- Test oculocephalic reflex (doll's eye manoeuvre).
- Test oculovestibular reflex (ear canal caloric stimulation).

IX, X Glossopharyngeal, Vagus

- Assess the patient's voice for hoarseness.
- Ask the patient to swallow and cough.
- Examine the palate for uvular displacement.
- Assess the soft palate movement by asking the patient to say 'ah'.
- Perform the gag reflex.

XI Accessory

- Examine for atrophy and asymmetry of the trapezius muscle.
- Ask the patient to shrug their shoulders.
- Turn the patient's head against resistance, inspect and palpate the sternocleidomastoid muscle.

XII Hypoglossal

- Listen to articulation.
- Inspect the patient's tongue for wasting or fasciculations.
- Ask the patient to protrude their tongue – The tongue will deviate to the affected side.

THE GLASGOW COMA SCALE EXAMINATION

Introduction and handwash

- Have the patient sitting up in the examination couch or chair.
- The Glasgow Coma Scale (GCS) Examination provides a reliable and objective way of recording the conscious level of the patient. Three types of responses (eye, verbal and motor) are independently assessed.
- Ask the patient whether they have any pain (if they are conscious).

Inspection

General

- Look at the patient as a whole (well/unwell; pain/pain free).
- Check the patient's prescription chart for medication (*i.e. sedation and analgesia*) that may alter the conscious level of the patient.

Specific

- Scoring system is used to monitor changes in the level of consciousness.
- The total score is the summation of the eye, verbal and motor responses.
- The range is from 3 (worst) to 15 (best).

Best Eye Response

- Spontaneously 4
- To speech 3
- To pain 2
- No response 1

Best Verbal Response

- Orientated 5
- Confused 4
- Inappropriate responses 3
- Inappropriate sounds 2
- No response 1

Best Motor Response

- Obeys commands 6
- Localise to pain 5
- Withdraws from pain 4
- Flexion (decorticate) to pain 3
- Extension (decerebrate) to pain 2
- No response 1

Please record the patient's

- Pupil size – 1–8 (mm),
- Pupil reaction – +: reacts, –: no reaction, c: closed eyes and
- Limb movement – Normal power, mild weakness, severe weakness, spastic flexion, extension and no response.
- It is important to document the patient's GCS and pupil size and reaction prior to intubation (Figure 8.1).

Thank the patient and wash hands.

Summarise and offer your differential diagnosis.

THE CEREBELLAR EXAMINATION

Cerebellar dysfunction is assessed by using the mnemonic: DANISH.

Dysdiadochokinesia:

- Ask the patient to rapidly pronate and supinate their hand on the opposite hand, repeat in other hand. They will have an inability to perform rapid alternating movements.

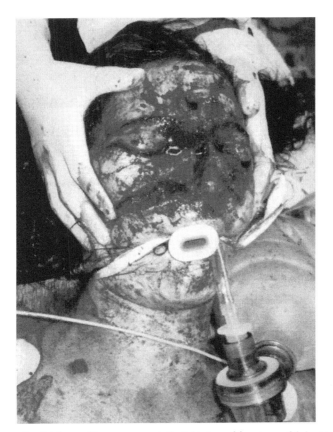

Figure 8.1 Unrestrained driver with severe craniofacial injury. (Courtesy of Johannesburg Hospital Trauma Unit.)

Ataxia:

- Assess for a broad-based unsteady gait with lumbering movements. The patient may demonstrate variable distance between steps and difficulty with turning.

Nystagmus:

- Assess for oscillating eye movements.

Intention tremor:

- Ask the patient to point from their nose to your finger. Ensure your finger is at arms length and then move finger to different places. As the patient's finger approaches your finger a tremor may be noticed or there may be evidence of past-pointing.

Staccato speech:

- Ask the patient to repeat 'British constitution' or 'baby hippopotamus'.

<u>Hy</u>potonia:

- Assess for reduced tone in the patient's upper and lower limbs.

THE GAIT EVALUATION

Walking – initiation, gait symmetrical, size of paces, posture, arms swing, turning, speed, fluency of stepping, stride length, distance between feet (base), inspect the patient's knees, pelvis and shoulders.

Inspect the patient's shoes.

Ask the patient to heel-to-toe walk (as if on a tight-rope), walk on their toes and heals.

Romberg test (to assess the dorsal columns of the spinal cord) – Ask the patient to stand with their feet together and ask the patient to close their eyes.

THE PERIPHERAL NERVOUS SYSTEM EXAMINATION (UPPER AND LOWER LIMBS)

Introduction and handwash

- Have the patient sitting up in the examination couch or chair.
- Expose the patient's upper and lower limbs.
- Ask the patient whether they have any pain.
- Remember the anatomy of the spinal cord tracts:
  - Descending pyramidal tract – Corticospinal tract (i.e. arm/leg weakness [UMN])
  - Descending extra-pyramidal tract – Rubrospinal/Vestibulospinal (i.e. ataxia)
  - Spinothalamic tract – Pain and temperature sensation
  - Dorsal columns – Light touch, proprioception and vibration sense
  - Autonomic pathways – Bladder and sexual function
- Remember the spinal nerve is a mixed nerve:
  - Sensory root
    Specific dermatomal sensory deficit (pain, temperature, light touch, joint position sense [JPS], vibration and co-ordination).
  - Motor root
    In LMN deficits, look for weakness, fasciculation, muscle wasting or loss of reflexes.

Inspection

General

- Look around bed for aids (walking, hearing).
- Look at the patient as a whole (well/unwell; pain/pain free).

Specific

- Inspect the patient's muscles for wasting, hypertrophy and involuntary movements (fasciculations, choreiform movements, tremor or jerks).
- Assess the patient's gait.
- Perform Romberg's test.

  - Ask the patient to stand with feet together, eyes open and hands by the sides. The patient should then close their eyes. Maintaining balance whilst standing relies on intact sensory pathways, sensorimotor integration centres and motor pathways.
  - The first stage (standing with the eyes open) demonstrates that at least one of the sensory pathways is intact.
  - In the second stage, the visual pathway is removed by closing the eyes. If the proprioceptive pathway is intact, balance will be maintained.
  - A positive Romberg test will demonstrate a sensory ataxia. This occurs with disruption in the dorsal columns of the spinal cord (*i.e. tabes dorsalis neurosyphilis*), disruption of the sensory nerves (*i.e. chronic inflammatory demyelinating polyradiculoneuropathy*) or when there is vestibular dysfunction.

Tone

- Ask the patient to relax and 'go floppy'.
- Upper limb – Roll arm in clock and counter clockwise directions.
- Lower limb – Roll leg and lift and release the patient's knee.

  - UMN lesions – 'Clasp knife' spasticity and 'lead pipe' rigidity.
  - Parkinson's disease – 'Cogwheel' rigidity.

- Assess for clonus.

Support the patient's flexed knee with one hand. Use your other hand to sharply dorsiflex the foot and sustain pressure. If positive, there will be a continued rhythmical beating of the foot.

Power

- Perform isometric and isotonic testing.
- Assess individual muscles groups and compare each side.
- Please record the *Medical Research Council (MRC) Grading of Power*

  - 5/5 Normal – Movement against gravity – full power
  - 4/5 Movement against specific gravity and resistance, but weaker than normal
  - 3/5 Movement against gravity
  - 2/5 Movement with gravity eliminated
  - 1/5 Visible contraction, but no movement
  - 0/5 No contraction

Upper limb function:

Movement	Root	Nerve	Muscle
Shoulder abduction	C5	Axillary	Deltoid
Elbow flexion	C5	Musculocutaneous	Biceps
Elbow flexion	C6	Radial	Brachioradialis
Elbow extension	C7	Radial	Triceps
Wrist extension	C6	Radial	Extensor carpi radialis longus
Finger extension	C7	Posterior interosseus	Extensor digitorum communis
Finger flexion	C8	Anterior interosseus	Flexor digitorum profundus (index)
Finger flexion	C8	Ulnar	Flexor digitorum profundus (ring + little)
Finger abduction	T1	Ulnar	Abductor digit minimi
Finger abduction	T1	Median	Abductor pollicis brevis

Cervical nerve root lesion in the upper limb:

Root	C5	C6	C7	C8	T1
Sensory loss	Lat. border upper arm to elbow	Lat. forearm, thumb and index finger	Middle finger, front and back of hand	Hypothenar eminence	Axilla
Pain distribution	As above medial scapula border	As above, especially, thumb and index finger	As above	As above Up to elbow	Shoulder, axilla to olecranon
Motor deficit	Deltoid Supraspinatus Infraspinatus	Biceps, brachioradialis, pronators and supinators of forearm	Triceps wrist extension wrist flexors Latissimus dorsi pectorialis major	Finger flexors and finger extensors	Small muscles of hand
Reflex arc	Biceps	Supinator	Triceps	Finger	None

Lower limb function:

Movement	Root	Nerve	Muscle
Hip flexion	L2/L3	Femoral	Iliopsoas
Hip adduction	L2/L3	Obturator	Adductors
Hip extension	L4/L5	Sciatic	Gluteus maximus
Knee flexion	L5/S1	Sciatic	Hamstrings
Knee extension	L3/L4	Femoral	Quadriceps
Ankle dorsiflexion	L4/L5	Deep peroneal	Tibialis anterior
Ankle eversion	L5/S1	Superficial peroneal	Peronei
Ankle plantar flexion	S1/S2	Tibial	Gastrocnemius
Big toe extension	L5	Deep peroneal	Extensor hallucis longus

Lumbar radiculopathy secondary to lumbar disc protrusions:

	L3/L4	L4/L5	L5/S1
%Disc	5%	45%	50%
Root	L4	L5	S1
Reflex	Knee		Ankle
Motor	Knee extension	Extensor hallucis longus, tibialis anterior (foot dorsiflexion)	Foot plantar flexion
Sensory	Medial calf	Lateral calf	Lateral foot
Pain	Anterior thigh	Posterior leg	Peroneus longus, ankle

Co-ordination

Upper limb function:

- Finger-nose test
  - Ask the patient to hold their arm outstretched and then touch the tip of their index finger to their nose and then to your index finger. Next, move your index finger in order for the patient to touch a new target.
- Rapid alternating hand movements
  - Ask the patient to simulate they are playing the piano.
  - Ask the patient to place their palms upwards. The patient should then tap the upward facing palm with their palmar and then doral aspect of their fingertips from the other hand.

Lower limb function:

- Heal-shin test
  - Ask the patient to raise one leg at the hip and place their heel of the flexed leg on their contralateral knee and then run their heel down the anterior surface of their shin towards their ankle. Repeat the process again in both lower limbs.
- Heel-toe test of gait
  - Ask the patient to walk in a straight line in order for the heel of one foot to be in contact with toes of their other foot. Ask the patient to walk 'heel-to-toe'.

Sensation

Fine touch function:

- Establish a baseline for fine touch (*i.e. sternal area*) before examining the limbs.
- Assess fine touch by using a small piece of cotton wool.
- Ask the patient to close their eyes and to respond when they are touched.
- Alter the timing of the stimulus so the patient does not anticipate the stimulus.
- Examine the spinal segments with an anatomical system (follow the dermatomal distribution).
- Compare this sensation on each of the patient's limbs for symmetry. The patient should also report the quality and quantity of this sensation (Figure 8.2).

Upper limb		Lower limb	
C5	Lateral arm	L1	Below inguinal ligament
C6	Thumb and index finger	L2	Middle thigh
C7	Middle finger	L3	Lower thigh
C8	Ring and small finger	L4	Medial leg and medial foot
T1	Medial arm	L5	Lateral leg and dorsal foot
		S1	Lateral foot

Pain function:

- Establish a baseline for sharpness (*i.e. sternal area*) before examining the limbs.
- Assess pain by using a dedicated disposable pin.
- Ask the patient to close their eyes and to respond when they are touched.
- Alter the timing of the stimulus so the patient does not anticipate the stimulus.
- Examine the spinal segments with an anatomical system (follow the dermatomal distribution).
- Compare this sensation on each of the patient's limbs for symmetry. The patient should also report the quality and quantity of this sensation.

Temperature function:

- Establish a baseline for temperature (*i.e. sternal area*) before examining the limbs.
- Assess temperature by using a cold and warmed tuning fork or plastic container.

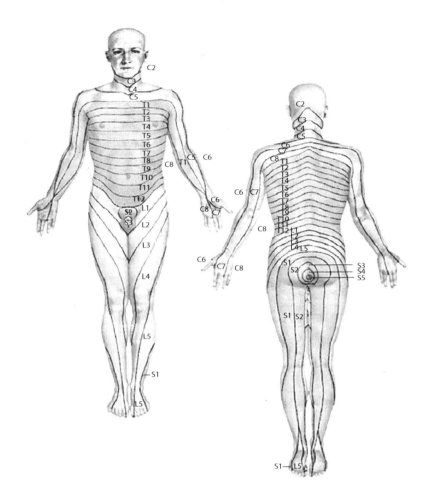

Figure 8.2 Dermatomal distributions.

- Ask the patient to close their eyes and to respond when they are touched.
- Alter the timing of the stimulus so the patient does not anticipate the stimulus.
- Examine the spinal segments with an anatomical system (follow the dermatomal distribution).
- Compare this sensation on each of the patient's limbs for symmetry. The patient should also report the quality and quantity of this sensation.

JPS function:

- Demonstrate the intended movement to the patient before examining the limbs.
- Assess JPS in the distal part of the limbs (distal interphalangeal joints [DIPJs] of the index finger and hallux).
- Ask the patient to close their eyes, move their distal phalanx up and down.
- Ask the patient to identify the direction of the movement.
- Compare this function on each of the patient's limbs for symmetry.

Vibration function:

- Establish a baseline for vibration (*i.e. over the sternum*) before examining the limbs.
- Assess vibration by using a tuning fork (128 Hz).
- Ask the patient to close their eyes and to respond when they are touched.
- Alter the timing of the stimulus so the patient does not anticipate the stimulus.
- In the upper limbs, use the interphalangeal joint (IPJ) of the forefinger, wrist, elbow or shoulder. In the lower limbs, use the big toes, ankle (medial malleolus), tibial tuberosity or iliac crest.
- Compare this sensation on each of the patient's limbs for symmetry.

Two-point discrimination function:

- Assess discrimination by using an opened paperclip.
- Ask the patient to close their eyes and to respond when they are touched.
- Alter the timing of the stimulus so the patient does not anticipate the stimulus.
- Apply the opened paperclip to the digits.
- Ask the patient if one or two stimuli are felt.

Reflexes

- Perform deep tendon and superficial reflexes. If the reflex is absent, you may be able to enhance the reflex with reinforcement.
- Ensure the patient is in a position of comfort with the limbs relaxed.
- Tap the tendon of the muscle with a tendon hammer and observe for muscle contraction.
- Please record the *Grading*:

  4+ Hyperactive with clonus
  3+ Hyperactive without clonus
  2+ Normal
  1+ Hypoactive
  0 Absent

Tendon reflex:

Upper limb	Lower limb
Biceps (C5, musculocutaneous nerve)	Patellar (L3–4, femoral nerve)
Brachioradialis (C6, radial nerve)	Achilles (S1–2, tibia nerve)
Triceps (C7, radial nerve)	

Other reflexes include:

- Finger jerks (C8)
- Hoffmann reflex – Hold the patient's middle finger (DIPJ) and briskly flick the patient's fingertip down and examine the patient's thumb for movement
- Pectoral reflex
- Deltoid reflex

- Plantar response – Apply blunt implement to the lateral border of the patient's sole. A normal reflex is plantar flexion of the hallux with flexion and adduction of the other toes
- Abdominal response
- Cremasteric reflex

Thank the patient and wash hands.

Summarise and offer your differential diagnosis.

THE MEDIAN NERVE EXAMINATION

Introduction and handwash

- Have the patient in a comfortable position on the examination couch or chair.
- Obtain adequate exposure.
- Ask the patient whether they have any pain.

Look

General

- Look around bed for aids (wrist splints).
- Look at the patient as a whole (well/unwell; pain/pain free).
- Look for signs of *endocrine causes* (acromegaly, myxoedema), *connective tissue disease (rheumatoid arthritis), fluid retention (congestive cardiac failure, pregnancy) and trauma.*

Specific

Inspect the following structures:

- Skin – Carpal tunnel decompression scars, pulp atrophy and cigarette burns.
- Muscle – Wasting of thenar eminence, flexors in the forearm, the short flexors, abductor and opponens of the thumb, the lumbricals to the index and middle finger.
- Bone – Simian thumb.

Feel

- Ask the patient whether they are in pain before you begin.
- Palpate for pain in the hand.
- Palpate the median nerve at the wrist (superficial site).
- Palpate sensation over the dorsal aspect of the patient's tip of index finger.
- Palpate over the thenar eminence.

Move

- Test the LOAF muscles (i.e. lateral 2 lumbricals, opponens pollicis, abductor pollicis brevis, and flexor pollicis brevis).

- Abductor pollicis brevis. Ask the patient to place their hand on the examination couch, palm facing up and to point their thumb to the ceiling. Ask the patient to resist you pushing their thumb down. Feel simultaneously for muscle contraction in the thenar eminence (Figure 8.3).
- Opposition (thumb to each finger).
- 'OK' sign test (tests flexor pollicis longus [FPL] thumb, flexor digitorum profundus [FDP] index finger; anterior interosseous branch of median nerve). Try to break the circle between their thumb and index finger (Figure 8.4).
- FPL – Hold the base of the thumb and ask the patient to bend the tip of their thumb.

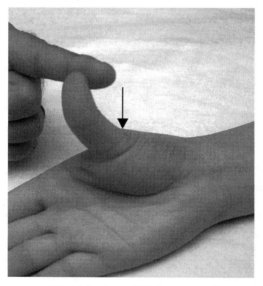

Figure 8.3 Testing the power of the abductor pollicis brevis supplied by the median nerve.

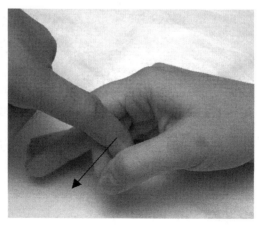

Figure 8.4 Test for flexor pollicis longus supplied by the anterior interosseus nerve.

- Test FDP – Fix the proximal interphalangeal joint [PIPJ] and isolate the DIPJ. Then ask the patient to bend the tip of their finger (Figure 8.5b).
- Test flexor digitorum superficialis (FDS) – Hold the other fingers down in extension to eliminate FDP and then ask the patient to flex their finger (Figure 8.5a).
- Ask the patient to make a fist (look for the '*Benediction sign*') and inspect the volar forearm for contraction of palmaris longus and flexor carpi radialis (make a tight fist and flex at wrist to contract forearm muscles).
- Ask the patient to flex their wrist and look for ulnar deviation/adduction (unopposed action of flexor carpi ulnaris [FCU] due to weak forearm flexors).
- Assess pronator teres (extend the patient's elbow and pronate against resistance). You may also assess this by shaking the patient's hand and ask them to push against you.

Special Tests

- *Functional assessment*
  - Power grip
  - Pincer grip (pick up a coin or key)
  - Button and unbutton shirt
  - Hold a pen and write
- *Tinel's sign* (percuss over the median nerve from the top of the forearm down to the centre of the palm and ask the patient if they feel paraesthesia over the median nerve distribution).
- *Phalen's test* (hold the patient's wrists in maximum flexion for >60 seconds and ask the patient if they feel paraesthesia over the median nerve distribution).

Complete the Median Nerve Examination

- Perform a full neurological assessment of the upper and lower limbs.
- Perform a full vascular examination of the upper and lower limbs.

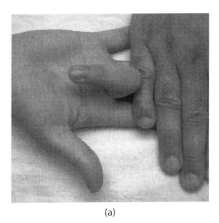 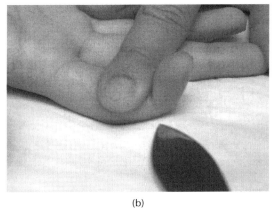

(a)   (b)

Figure 8.5 Testing the (a) flexor digitorum superficialis and (b) flexor digitorum profundus.

- Examine the joint above (shoulder and cervical spine).
- Assess the impact of the joint condition on the patient's life.
- Request nerve conduction studies.
- Consider imaging of the cervical spine (radiographs, magnetic resonance imaging [MRI] scan).
- Assess the patient's fitness for surgery.

Thank the patient and wash hands.

Summarise and offer your differential diagnosis.

THE RADIAL NERVE EXAMINATION

Introduction and handwash

- Have the patient in a comfortable position on the examination couch or chair.
- Obtain adequate exposure.
- Ask the patient whether they have any pain.

Look

General

- Look around bed for aids (wrist splints).
- Look at the patient as a whole (well/unwell; pain/pain free).

Specific

Inspect the following structures:

- Skin – Scars, pulp atrophy, cigarette burns.
- Muscle – Wasting of posterior forearm muscles (extensors).
- Bone – Wrist drop and fractures of the humeral shaft.
- Ask the patient to place their hands behind their head and check the elbows for scars (head radius fracture) and wasting of triceps muscles.
- Ask the patient to lift their hand off the examination couch and inspect for a wrist drop.

Feel

- Ask the patient whether they are in pain before you begin.
- Palpate for pain in the hand.
- Palpate over the anatomical snuffbox.
- Palpate over the first dorsal web space.
- Test sensation over the back of the forearm.

Move

- Test extension of the triceps muscle (high lesions).
- Test brachioradialis (flex the elbow in mid-prone position against resistance).

- Test supinator (extend the elbow and supinate against resistance – test this by holding their hand with your opposite hand, i.e. grip their right hand with your left hand and grip their left hand with your right hand). Ask them to push against you.
- Ask them to cock their wrist back against resistance (wrist extension).
- Test finger extension (ask the patient to keep their fingers straight and stop you from bending their fingers).
- Examine extensor pollicis longus (EPL) by performing the *retropulsion test* – ask the patient to put their hand on the examination couch, palm down and lift their thumb into the air, against resistance (see Figure 8.6).

Special tests

- *Functional assessment*
  - Power grip
  - Pincer grip (pick up a coin or key)
  - Button and unbutton shirt
  - Hold a pen and write

Complete the radial nerve examination

- Perform a full neurological assessment of the upper and lower limbs.
- Perform a full vascular examination of the upper and lower limbs.
- Examine the joint above (shoulder and cervical spine).
- Assess the impact of the joint condition on the patient's life.
- Request nerve conduction studies. Consider a radiograph of the humerus and radiograph and/or MRI scan of the cervical spine.
- Assess the patient's fitness for surgery.

Thank the patient and wash hands.

Summarise and offer your differential diagnosis.

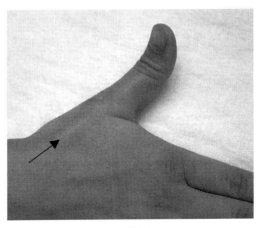

Figure 8.6 Testing the integrity of extensor pollicis longus.

THE ULNAR NERVE EXAMINATION

Introduction and handwash

- Have the patient in a comfortable position on the examination couch or chair.
- Obtain adequate exposure.
- Ask the patient whether they have any pain.

Look

General

- Look around bed for aids (wrist splints).
- Look at the patient as a whole (well/unwell; pain/pain free).

Specific

Inspect the following structures:

Dorsum surface:

- Skin – Pulp atrophy, scars, cigarette burns, brittle nails.
- Muscle – Wasting first dorsal web space, interosseous, dorsal guttering (Figure 8.7).
- Bone – 'claw hand'.

Palmar surface:

- Skin – as above.
- Muscle – Wasting hypothenar eminence, wasting medial forearm muscles.
- Bone – Ask the patient to lay their hand flat down on the table to assess whether, or not, any fixed flexion deformity (FFD) is fixed ('table-top test').

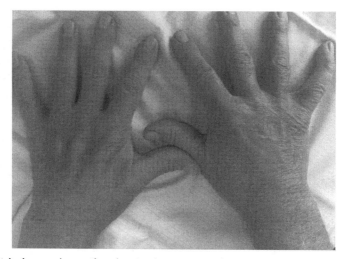

Figure 8.7 Intrinsic muscle wasting due to ulnar neuropathy.

Upper limbs:

Ask the patient to place their hands behind their head. Check the elbows for scars around the medial epicondyle/forearm/wrist and check elbow for cubitus valgus (tardy ulnar syndrome).

Feel

- Ask the patient whether they are in pain before you begin.
- Palpate along the ulnar nerve behind the patient's medial epicondyle and over the wrist joint.
- Test the sensation over the tip of the little and ring fingers (volar surface).
- Turn hands over and test the dorsal cutaneous branch of ulnar nerve (given off proximal to the wrist).

Move

- First dorsal interosseous – Resisted abduction of index finger and palpate the first dorsal web space.
- Abductor digiti minimi – Repeat the same with the little finger.
- Finger adductors:
  - Palmar interossei – Hold a piece of paper in between the patient's fingers and ask them to try to stop you from pulling the paper away.
- Finger abductors:
  - Doral interossei – Ask the patient to spread fingers apart and stop you from pushing them together.
  - Ask the patient to put their hands together palms up and little fingers touching. Ask patient to push the little fingers together.
- Ulnar 1/2 FDP – Ask the patient to bend the tip of little finger at DIPJ.
- FCU and ulnar 1/2 FDP – Ask the patient to make a fist (grip hard with wrist flexion). Examine for muscle contraction.
- FCU (wrist flexion and ulnar deviation at the wrist) – Ask patient to flex and adduct their wrist. Note when FCU is paralysed – Flexion at the wrist joint will result in abduction.

Special tests

- *Functional assessment*
  - Power grip
  - Pincer grip (pick up a coin or key)
  - Button and unbutton shirt
  - Hold a pen and write
- *Froment's sign (Figure 8.8).* Ask the patient to grasp a piece of paper between their thumb and index finger (using both hands). Try to pull paper away. Note if there

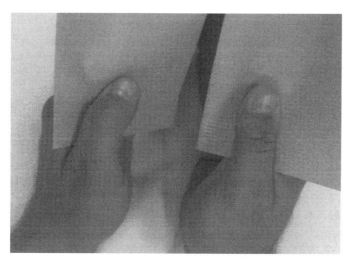

Figure 8.8 Froment's sign tests the adductor pollicis. Patient is asked to hold a piece of paper in a side pinch between the thumb and the index finger. The examiner attempts to pull the paper out. Due to weakness of the adductor pollicus the patient will compensate by flexing the FPL that is supplied by the anterior interosseous nerve.

is flexing of the terminal phalanx as you pull away. This test assesses adductor pollicis: in ulnar nerve palsy, the FPL flexes the IPJ to compensate.

- *Tinel's percussion test* over Guyon's canal and at elbow.
- *Elbow flexion test* (patient flexes both their elbows and holds them in close to body. Wait 1 minute to see if the patient complains of paraesthesia).

Complete the ulnar nerve examination

- Perform a full neurological assessment of the upper and lower limbs.
- Perform a full vascular examination of the upper and lower limbs.
- Examine the joint above (shoulder and cervical spine).
- Assess the impact of the joint condition on the patient's life.
- Request nerve conduction studies. Consider a radiograph and/or MRI scan of the cervical spine.
- Assess the patient's fitness for surgery.

Thank the patient and wash hands.

Summarise and offer your differential diagnosis.

CHAPTER 9: TRUNK AND THORAX

LUMP IN THE BREAST: HISTORY TAKING

You are a junior doctor on Miss Woo's breast team. Miss Woo has asked you to clerk a new patient in the outpatient clinic. The general practitioner (GP) referral letter is attached. After you have taken the history, you will be asked to present it to one of the examiners as though he/she were the consultant.

Dr R Van der Berg

76 Turlington Terrace
London

The Consultant Breast Surgeon
King George's Hospital
London

Re: Cornelia Tristan-Davies, 45 Bleinham Square, London
Dear Doctor
I would be grateful if you could see this 56-year-old lady who came to us with a lump in her left breast.

Best wishes
Yours sincerely
Dr K Sanderson (locum)

Take a standard focused surgical history (presenting complaint, history presenting complaint, past medical history, drug history and allergies, social history, family history, systemic enquiry), but in particular enquire about the following:

- Age
- Lump site, single or multiple
- Lump onset, growth rate, variations with menstrual cycle
- Presence or absence of pain – Cyclical
- Change in breast size or shape
- Skin and nipple changes
- Discharge – Serous, serosanguinous, green, bloody, milk
- Temperature/fevers
- Weight loss
- Bone or abdominal pain
- Arm swelling (lymphoedema)
- Previous radiation or surgery – E.g. radiotherapy for Hodgkin's disease
- Menstrual history – Menarche, menopause, oral contraceptive pill (OCP), hormone replacement therapy (HRT)
- Obstetric history – Breast feeding and complications, parity previous mammograms, screening
- Family history – Breast, bowel, ovarian carcinoma (BRCA 1/2)
- Symptoms of possible metastatic disease – Other lumps (e.g. axilla), breathlessness, backache, headaches, tiredness, anorexia, weight loss etc.

How do you assess breast lumps in clinic?

- *Triple assessment*
  - History and physical examination

- Radiology – Mammography or ultrasound scan (USS) (in younger patients)
- Pathology – Fine needle aspiration cytology (FNAC) or core biopsy

What do you know about the breast screening programme?

- Patients on GP practice age range 50–70 years are invited
- Every 3 years
- Mammogram of each breast
- Set up in 1988 by the UK Department of Health

What are the common differentials for a malignant breast lump?

- Fibroadenoma
- Cyst
- Abscess
- Lipoma
- Fat necrosis
- Radiotherapy

BREAST: EXAMINATION

The opening

- Introduce yourself to the patient (permission)
- Ask for a nurse chaperone
- Obtain consent
- Ensure adequate privacy, patient comfort and exposure (position at 45°)
- Ask whether there is any pain present
- Wash hands

Inspection

From foot of bed and patient's right-hand side.

- General and peripheral stigmata – Jaundice, anaemia, cyanosis, clubbing, oedema, lymphadenopathy (JACCOL), cachexia
- Focussed inspection – Asymmetry, nipple changes, scars, skin changes, skin tethering, peau d'orange, lumps and swellings, effects of radiotherapy, lymphoedema
  - 'Slow arm abduction' (accentuates asymmetry)
  - 'Hands behind head' (inspect axillae – Scars, swellings, radiotherapy; inframammary folds – Lift each breast)
  - 'Hands on hips and press in' (tenses pectorals and accentuates asymmetry, deep structure tethering and absence in radical mastectomy)
  - 'Forward lean' (accentuate abnormalities in large pendulous breasts)
  - Inspect the back (evidence of latissimus dorsi reconstruction)
  - Inspect the abdomen (evidence of transverse rectus abdominis flap (TRAM) reconstruction)

Palpation

- Begin with unaffected breast first (redress other breast to preserve dignity)
- 'Any tenderness?'
- 'Hand behind head and tilt to contralateral side' (breast then lies flat on chest wall)
- Palpate seven areas in each breast for lumps (four quadrants; axillary tail of Spence; nipple-areolar complex; inframammary fold)
- In clinical practice, you should also palpate the retro-areolar tissue to try and express nipple discharge (but unlikely to be required in the Membership of the Royal College of Surgeons Objective Structured Clinical Examination [MRCS OSCE])
- Palpate in the axilla for lymph nodes (four walls and apex)
- Supraclavicular lymph nodes

Any lump?

- 'Press hands into hips' for pectoralis contraction and palpate for fixity and tethering.
- Define lump characteristics.

Surgical sequelae post-mastectomy?

- Sensation in the armpit and lateral chest wall (intercostobrachial nerve T2)
- Scapula winging (long thoracic nerve C5, C6, C7)

The closure

- Physical examination of the chest (lungs), back, abdomen (hepatomegaly), neurological system (brain metastasis)
- Assess fitness for surgery
- Thank the patient
- Wash hands
- Summarise and offer differential diagnosis

MIDLINE STERNOTOMY SCAR: EXAMINATION

The opening

- Introduce yourself to the patient (permission)
- Ask for a nurse chaperone
- Obtain consent
- Ensure adequate privacy, patient comfort and exposure (position at 45°)

- Ask whether any pain is present
- Wash hands

Inspection

From foot of bed and patient's right-hand side.

- General and peripheral stigmata – Oxygen and ventilation adjuncts, electrocardiogram (ECG) monitor, pulse oximeter, anaemia and cyanosis (cardiorespiratory disease), tar stains, splinter haemorrhages (infective endocarditis), amputations (peripheral vascular disease [PVD]), venous graft harvesting scars (long saphenous vein, radial artery).
- Focussed inspection – Chest scars (midline sternotomy, drains, pacemaker, implantable cardiac defibrillator [ICD]), chest wall movements (asymmetry – lung problem).

Palpation

- Begin with hands – Warmth, pulse
- Palpate sternotomy scar (malunion)
- Thrills
- Apex beat
- Other scars (pacemaker, ICD – Usually left lateral infraclavicular area)

Auscultation

- Apex beat, left lower sternal edge, left and right parasternal edge at second intercostals space (murmurs, mechanical valves)
- Lung bases (heart failure)

The closure

- Physical examination of the respiratory system (lungs), peripheral vascular system, abdomen (abdominal aortic aneurysm [AAA]).
- Observation chart (heart rate [HR], blood pressure [BP], temperature, respiratory rate [RR], oxygen saturation)
- Urine dipstick (haematuria – Infective endocarditis)
- ECG
- Chest x-ray (CXR)
- Thank the patient
- Wash hands
- Summarise and offer differential diagnosis

Can you tell how many grafts have been used in a coronary artery bypass graft (CABG) procedure by the length of the harvest skin scar? Why?

- No
- Harvested vessels are only used for CABG if they are of adequate calibre.
- The internal mammary artery may have been used for CABG.

CHANGE IN BOWEL HABIT: HISTORY TAKING

You are a junior doctor on Mr. Khan's general surgery team. Mr. Khan has asked you to clerk a new patient in the outpatient clinic. The GP referral letter is attached. After you have taken the history, you will be asked to present it to one of the examiners as though he or she were the consultant. He or she will then ask you for your differential diagnosis, what signs you would look for on examination and what investigations you would request.

Drs A Goldberg, S Patel, and P Carter

21 The Avenue
London

The Consultant Surgeon
St John's Hospital
London

Re: Olivier de Bourbon, 143 Daffodil Close, Surrey
Dear Doctor
This professional 41-year-old gentleman is describing some changes in bowel habit, diarrhoea, and an episode of bleeding.

Best wishes
Yours sincerely
Stuart Patel

Take a standard focused surgical history (presenting complaint, history presenting complaint, past medical history, drug history and allergies, social history, family history, systemic enquiry), but in particular enquire about the following:

- Nature of bowel habit – Diarrhoea, constipation
- Tenesmus
- Per rectum (PR) bleeding – Bright red, mixed in with stool, dark
- Mucous
- Weight loss
- Duration
- Time course and progression
- Risk factors – Family history

Differential diagnosis

- Colon cancer
- Rectal cancer
- Caecal cancer

- Diverticular disease
- Inflammatory bowel disease (IBD)
- Polyp
- Haemorrhoids
- Skin tags

Signs to look for on examination:

- General physical status of patient (cachexia, JACCOL)
- Check for peripheral stigmata of colorectal disease such as koilonychia (iron deficiency anaemia), conjunctival pallor, angular stomatitis (Crohn's disease), aphthous ulcers (Crohn's disease), lip/mouth pigmentation (Peutz–Jegher's syndrome)
- Abdominal examination checking for masses, ascites, hepatosplenomegaly
- Digital rectal examination (DRE) and proctoscopy
- Rigid sigmoidoscopy

Investigations

- Faecal occult blood (caecal malignancy)
- Blood tests
  - Haematology – Full blood count (FBC) (anaemia – malignancy, IBD, polyps), white cell count (WCC) (IBD)
  - Biochemistry – U+Es (dehydration), liver function tests (LFTs) (liver metastases), C-reactive protein (CRP)
  - Tumour markers – Carcinoembryonic antigen (CEA), CA19-9

Radiology

- Abdominal x-ray (AXR) (mass, IBD)
- Barium enema (mass, polyps, IBD)

Endoscopy

- Flexible sigmoidoscopy (suspected distal colon malignancy)
- Colonoscopy (suspected caecal malignancy, IBD)

If cancer is suspected, what is your subsequent management plan likely to entail?

- Referral to multi-disciplinary team (MDT)
- Computed tomography (CT) chest, abdomen, pelvis (staging)
- Magnetic resonance (MR) rectum (in cases specifically of rectal cancer for operative planning)
- USS liver (in suspected liver metastasis)
- Patient and family discussions, consent for treatment
- Pre-operative anaesthetic assessments

ABDOMEN: EXAMINATION

The opening

- Introduce yourself to the patient (permission)
- Ask for a nurse chaperone
- Obtain consent
- Ensure adequate privacy, patient comfort and exposure (lie flat with one pillow)
- Ask the patient whether they have any pain
- Wash hands

Inspection

From foot of bed and patient's right-hand side.

- General and peripheral stigmata – Oxygen and ventilation adjuncts, intravenous infusion (IVI), JACCOL, leukonychia (hypoalbuminaemia), koilonychia (iron deficiency anaemia), palmar erythema (liver disease), Dupuytren's contracture (liver disease), liver flap, pulse (tachycardia, atrial fibrillation [AF]), aphthous ulcers (Crohn's disease), mouth pigmentation (Peutz–Jegher's syndrome), gynaecomastia (liver disease), spider naevi (portal hypertension), supraclavicular nodes (Virchow).
- Focussed inspection – Abdomen moving freely with respiration, distension, scars, fistulae, pulsatility, lift head off bed (accentuates abdominal herniae), stomas, tubes (suprapubic catheter, nephrostomy), drains.

Palpation

- Palpate the tenderest point last. *You must look at the patient's face at all* times as you superficially palpate the quadrants and central area for tenderness and obvious masses.
- Deep palpation of nine abdominal areas for masses.
- Liver – Palpate from the right iliac fossa (RIF) on deep inspiration towards right upper quadrant (RUQ) (hepatomegaly).
- Spleen – Palpate from the RIF on deep inspiration towards left upper quadrant (LUQ). To accentuate, repeat with patient rolled to their right side (splenomegaly).
- Kidneys – Bimanual balloting (renal tumour, polycystic kidneys).
- AAA – Expansile, pulsatile mass in the epigastrium.
- Groins – Cough impulse at deep ring (hernia).
- Ankles (oedema).

Percussion

- Percussion tenderness (peritonitis)
- Liver size (hepatomegaly)

- Spleen size (splenomegaly)
- Shifting dullness (ascites)

Auscultation

- Bowel sounds
- Renal bruits
- Venous hums
- Friction rubs
- Femoral artery bruits

The closure

- Physical examination of external genitalia
- DRE
- Observation chart (HR, BP, temperature)
- Fluid balance chart
- Urine dipstick (haematuria, urinary tract infection [UTI])
- Stool chart
- AXR
- Thank the patient
- Wash hands
- Summarise and offer differential diagnosis

How would you describe this scar?

- Old or recent
- Well healed or poorly healed
- Trophic abnormalities – Atrophic, hypertrophic, keloid
- Presence or absence of infection
- Associated complications – Incisional hernia
- Other scars – Drain sites, stoma sites, laparoscopic ports

ABDOMINAL MASS: EXAMINATION

The opening

- Introduce yourself to the patient (permission)
- Ask for a nurse chaperone
- Obtain consent
- Ensure adequate privacy, patient comfort and exposure (lie flat with one pillow)
- Ask the patient whether they have any pain
- Wash hands

Inspection, palpation, percussion, auscultation

- Site
- Scars overlying it (e.g. renal transplant)
- Size
- Shape
- Surface – Regular/irregular
- Edge – Regular/irregular
- Tenderness
- Temperature
- Consistency
- Can you get above/below it?
- Gently pinch skin over it
- Lift head off the bed (tense the rectus sheath) to determine mobility/fixity of mass
- Cough impulse
- Reducibility/compressibility
- Fluctuance
- Pulsatility and expansility
- Does it move with respiration?
- Can it be ballotted?
- Percuss the lump
- Auscultate over the lump
- Palpate for regional lymph nodes (inguinal and axillary)
- Neurovascular status

The closure

- Thank the patient
- Wash hands
- Summarise and offer differential diagnosis

HEPATOMEGALY AND SPLENOMEGALY

You palpate an enlarged liver. Can you describe it?

- Extension distance beneath the costal margin (cm/finger breadths)
- Percuss upper liver border of the liver (to assess whether it is pushed down by lung hyperexpansion)
- Consistency – Soft, firm, hard, craggy (cirrhosis, tumour)
- Liver edge – Smooth, nodular (cirrhosis, tumour)

- Liver tenderness (hepatitis)
- Liver pulsatility
- Presence or absence of a Reidel's lobe

What might be causing it?

Physiological:

- Riedel's lobe
- Hyperexpanded chest (liver ptosis)

Pathological:

- Infection – Virus (viral hepatitis, Epstein–Barr virus [EBV], cytomegalovirus [CMV], human immunodeficiency virus [HIV]), bacteria (tuberculosis [TB], abscess), protozoa (malaria, hydatid, amoebiasis, schistosomiasis)
- Neoplasia – Benign (hepatoma), malignant (hepatocellular carcinoma [HCC], cholangiocarcinoma, metastases, lymphoma, myeloproliferative disease)
- Vascular – Congestive cardiac failure [CCF]
- Metabolic – Alcohol (fatty liver, cirrhosis), Wilson's, haemochromatosis, saroidosis, amyloidosis, Gaucher's disease
- Other – Cysts

How do you distinguish the spleen from the left kidney clinically?

- Spleen descends towards RIF, left kidney descends towards left iliac fossa (LIF).
- Kidneys are ballotable, the spleen is not.
- It might be possible to palpate above the left kidney but not the spleen.
- Spleen has a palpable notch, kidneys do not.
- Spleen is usually dull to percussion but the left kidney may be resonant due to overlying bowel.
- Spleen may have a friction rub, kidneys do not.

You palpate an enlarged spleen. What might be causing it?

- Infection – Virus (EBV, CMV, HIV), bacteria (typhoid, typhus, TB, sepsis, bacterial endocarditis), protozoa (malaria, schistosomiasis, kala-azar).
- Neoplasia – Benign (haemolytic anaemias, pernicious anaemia, ITP, sickle cell disease), malignant (myeloproliferative, lymphoproliferative disorders).
- Vascular – Portal hypertension.
- Metabolic – Amyloidosis, rheumatoid arthritis (Felty's syndrome), Gaucher's disease, systemic lupus erythematosus (SLE), sarcoidosis.
- Other – Cysts.

What might cause both the liver and spleen to be enlarged?

- Portal hypertension
- Myeloproliferative disorders
- Lymphoproliferative disorders

CHRONIC LIVER DISEASE

What are the classical stigmata of chronic liver disease?

- Hands – Leukonychia (hypoalbuminaemia), clubbing, palmar erythema, Dupuytren's contracture, bruising (coagulopathy), liver flap (encephalopathy), pruritus/scratch marks (accumulation of bile salts in the skin).
- Face – Jaundice (hyperbilirubinaemia), scratch marks, spider naevi (portal hypertension), foetor hepaticus.
- Chest – Gynaecomastia (oestrogen metabolism dysfunction), loss of body hair, spider naevi (portal hypertension), bruising, pectoral muscle wasting.
- Abdomen – Signs of portal hypertension (hepatosplenomegaly, ascites, caput medusae), testicular atrophy.
- Legs – Oedema (hypoalbuminaemia), muscle wasting, bruising.

STOMA: EXAMINATION

Common stomas include ileostomy, colostomy, ileal conduit, nephrostomy, urostomy tracheostomy.

The opening

- Introduce yourself to the patient (permission)
- Ask for a nurse chaperone
- Obtain consent
- Ensure adequate privacy, patient comfort and exposure (lie flat with one pillow)
- Ask whether any pain is present
- Wash hands

Inspection

From foot of bed and patient's right-hand side.

- Site – Which quadrant, is it well sited? (away from bony prominences, scars, skin folds)
- Scars – Previous surgery and stomas
- Contents – Liquid faeces, formed faeces, urine
- Morphology – Spout (ileostomy) or flush (colostomy)
- Lumen – Single (end stoma) or double (loop stoma)
- Loop stoma – Presence of a bridge (a newly formed stoma), identify afferent limb (produces stool output and is usually larger and more caudally placed to prevent spill-over into efferent limb), identify efferent limb (allows passage of flatus and mucous discharge from defunctioned distal bowel and is usually smaller and more cephalically placed)
- State of the stoma (ischaemia/necrosis, ulceration, stenosis)
- Surrounding skin – Excoriation and erythema (poorly fitting bag)
- Parastomal hernia (lift head off bed and cough)
- Prolapse or retraction

- Mucocutaneous separation
- Output – High, e.g. in ileostomy

Palpation

- Digital stomal exam – Offer to insert a finger into the stoma to check stoma patency and for stenosis (and ensure bag is re-applied).
- Illuminate stomal tract – Shine a light down into the stoma to check the mucosa is healthy.

Auscultation

- Bowel sounds

The closure

- Inspection of perineum for scars and presence of anal opening
- Complete examination of abdomen
- Assess stoma position during sitting, lying and standing
- Thank the patient
- Wash hands
- Summarise and offer differential diagnosis (Figures 9.1 through 9.4)

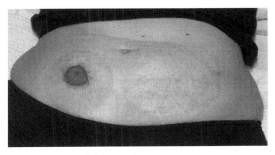

Figure 9.1 Spouted ileostomy in the right iliac fossa.

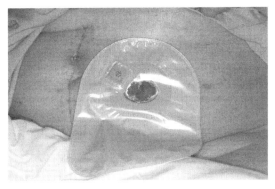

Figure 9.2 A colostomy in the left iliac fossa.

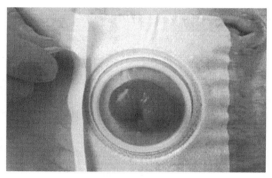

Figure 9.3 The usual long-term backing ('stomahesive') and flange, onto which the bag is being placed.

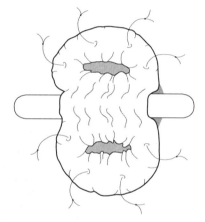

Figure 9.4 Temporary (loop) colostomy opened over a rod, and immediate suture of the colon wall to surrounding skin (alternatively, a skin bridge is used).

GROIN: EXAMINATION

The opening

- Introduce yourself to the patient (permission)
- Ask for a nurse chaperone
- Obtain consent
- Ensure adequate privacy, patient comfort and exposure (ask the patient to stand up and get full exposure of the groin, genitalia and abdomen. However, be prepared to be flexible depending on the patient's mobility)
- Ask whether any pain is present
- Wash hands.

N.B. Each time you ask the patient to cough, there should be a precise purpose (examiners will be watching how many times you make the patient cough and at which stage).

Inspection

- Lumps in the groin – Define its characteristics
- Scars (especially overlying any lumps)
- *Cough 1* – Look away and cough (inspect superficial ring of affected side for a cough impulse)
- *Cough 2* – Look away and cough (inspect superficial ring of contralateral side)

Palpation

Stand to patient's side with one hand on their back and the other hand on the lump itself.

- Any pain?
- Can you get above the lump? (If you cannot, it is likely to be a groin swelling and you should proceed as below. If you can get above the lump, it is likely to be a scrotal lump).
- Site – Key landmarks (anterior superior iliac spine [ASIS], pubic tubercle, the interposed inguinal ligament, femoral artery pulsation), relations to pubic tubercle (femoral vs. inguinal hernia).
- Lump characteristics.
- *Cough 3* – Expansile cough impulse.
- Reducibility – Ask the patient 'to push it back in if possible' (direct course: direct hernia, oblique course: indirect hernia).
- *Cough 4* – Place one finger on pubic tubercle and ask the patient to cough again (note the relation of lump to the pubic tubercle as it protrudes).

  - Above and medial to the pubic tubercle = inguinal hernia
  - Below and lateral to the pubic tubercle = femoral hernia

- *Cough 5* – Deep ring occlusion test: place one hand on the deep inguinal ring, above a point half way between the pubic tubercle and the ASIS, and then ask the patient to look away and cough (if the lump is controlled then the inguinal hernia is indirect).

Auscultation

- Bowel sounds – Viability of bowel

The closure

- Examination of contralateral groin
- Examination of genitalia – Coincidental hydrocoele, varicocele
- Examination of regional lymph nodes

- Full history
- Examination of the abdomen
- Digital rectal examination
- Assess fitness for surgery
- Thank the patient
- Wash hands
- Summarise and offer differential diagnosis

So you have found a lump in the groin – what do you think it is?

(This is best tackled anatomically with pathologies related to each layer.)

The differentials include

- Skin – Sebaceous cyst
- Subcutaneous tissues – Lipoma, fibroma
- Lymphatics – Inguinal lymphadenopathy
- Bowel – Inguinal, femoral hernia
- Vein – Saphena varix
- Artery – Femoral artery aneurysm
- Nerve – Neuroma, neurofibroma
- Spermatic cord – Lipoma of the cord, encysted hydrocoele of cord
- Testis/Scrotum – Ectopic testis
- Muscle – Benign/malignant tumour
- Psoas sheath – Psoas abscess, psoas bursa

EXTERNAL MALE GENITALIA: EXAMINATION

The opening

- Introduce yourself to the patient (permission)
- Ask for a nurse chaperone
- Obtain consent
- Ensure adequate privacy, patient comfort and exposure (ask the patient to stand up and get full exposure of the groin, genitalia and abdomen. However, be prepared to be flexible depending on the patient's mobility)
- Ask the patient whether they have any pain
- Wash hands

Inspection

- Lumps in the groin – Look away and cough
- Scars (including posterior aspect of scrotum)

Palpation

- Any pain?
- Can you get above the lump? (If you can get above the lump, it is likely to be a scrotal lump and you should proceed as below. If you cannot, it is likely to be a groin swelling.)
- Relations to testis – Assess whether the lump is separable from the testis
- Lump characteristics
- Relations to scrotal skin and scrotal skin pathology
- Transillumination – Bright (hydrocoele, epididymal cyst)
- Cough impulse – Look away and cough (indirect hernia)
- Examine contralateral side
- Examine the patient in the standing position to avoid missing a varicocele

The closure

- Take a full history
- Examination of the abdomen
- Digital rectal examination
- Assess fitness for surgery
- Thank the patient
- Wash hands
- Summarise and offer differential diagnosis

CHAPTER 10: VASCULAR

Model for a vascular history

Peripheral vascular system (upper and lower limbs): Examination

Venous system: Examination for varicose veins

Ulcer: Examination

MODEL FOR A VASCULAR HISTORY

Introduction

- Set the stage
    - Welcome the patient. Ensure comfort and privacy.
    - Know and use the patient's name. Introduce and identify yourself.
- Set the agenda
    - Begin with open-ended questions to ascertain the patient's perspective.
    - Encourage the consultations with silences and non-verbal and verbal cues.
    - Focus by paraphrasing and summarising.

Personal information

- Name, age, occupation and ethnic origin.

Presenting complaint (in the patient's own words)

History of presenting complaint

- System specific

Cardiac

- Angina – Location, time, mode on onset, severity, nature, progression, quantity, quality, frequency, duration, relieving and exacerbating factors, associated symptoms, radiation
- Dyspnoea – Including paroxysmal nocturnal, at rest and effort
- Orthopnoea
- Palpitations
- Headaches and dizziness
- Oedema (pulmonary, peripheral)

Peripheral Vascular

- Limb pain – Location, time, mode of onset, severity, nature, progression, quantity, quality, frequency, duration, relieving and exacerbating factors, associated symptoms, radiation
- Deformity
- Swelling
- Stiffness
- Amputations and ulceration
- Limb neurology weakness, paraesthesia
- Reduced range of movement
- Effects on function
- Walking distance

- **Risk factors** – Smoking, hypertension, diabetes, hypercholesterolemia, family history of atherosclerosis, diet
- **Investigations and treatment (medical, endovascular and surgical)**

Past medical, surgical and anaesthetic history

Medication, Allergies and Immunisations

Family history

Social history

- Marital status
- Occupation and exposures
- Smoking history
- Alcohol consumption

- Diet
- Illicit drug use
- Living accommodation
- Recent travel history

System Review

- General/Constitutional
- Skin/Breast
- Eyes/Ears/Nose/Mouth/Throat
- Respiratory
- Gastrointestinal
- Genitourinary
- Musculoskeletal
- Neurological
- Psychiatrical
- Immunologic/Lymphatic/Endocrine

Thank the patient

Summation

PERIPHERAL VASCULAR SYSTEM (UPPER AND LOWER LIMBS): EXAMINATION

Introduction and handwash

Start the examination with the patient in supine position with a pillow under their head for support. The patient's limbs (upper and lower) and chest should be fully exposed.

Ask the patient whether they have any pain.

Inspection

General

- Look around bed for aids, oxygen or medication (glyceryl trinitrate [GTN] spray).
- Look at the patient as a whole (well/unwell; pain/pain free; shortness of breath, cyanosis and obesity).

Specific

Upper limbs and Trunk

- Skin and nails – Tar staining, clubbing, brittle nails, splinter haemorrhages, vasculitic changes, pulp atrophy, digital colour changes/cyanosis, pale palmar creases, ulceration, gangrene and amputations

- Scars – Arm, neck (endarterectomy), chest (midline sternotomy), axilla (axillobifemoral bypass grafts), abdomen (laparotomy for abdominal aortic aneurysm [AAA])
- Horner's syndrome
- Muscle – Wasting

Lower limbs (Figure 10.1)

- Skin and nails – Nail changes for friability or dystrophic changes, skin colour, ulceration, gangrene, digital amputations/tissue loss, changes of coincidental venous disease, oedema (often due to dependency), hair loss and venous guttering.
- Scars (vein harvest, reconstruction procedures, grafts/flaps for soft tissue cover of ulcers and areas of tissue loss). Look for scars in the groin (exposure of common femoral artery).
- Muscles – Wasting (often due to disuse atrophy), loss of prominence of extensor tendons on the dorsum of foot (oedema).
- Don't forget to examine between the toes.

Palpation (ask the patient whether they are in pain before you begin)

Upper limbs

- Temperature of the upper limbs (with the back of the hand)
- Assess for the capillary refill time
- Palpate the radial pulses for rate and rhythm. Moreover, assess for radial, radio-radial delay, collapsing pulse
- Palpate the brachial pulse
- Assess the patient's blood pressure in both upper limbs
- Palpate the axillary artery in axilla
- Palpate the subclavian artery (subclavian aneurysm, post-stenotic dilatation)
- Palpate the carotid pulses for rate, rhythm and character
- Palpate the superficial temporal artery
- Palpate for a cervical rib

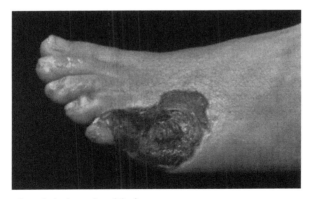

Figure 10.1 Severe chronic ischaemia with dry gangrene.

Lower limbs

- Temperature of the lower limbs (with the back of the hand).
- Assess for pitting oedema.
- Assess for capillary refill time.
- Palpate the abdomen for an *abdominal aortic pulse.*
- Palpate for a *femoral pulse* – Midway between the anterior superior iliac spine (ASIS) and the symphysis pubis at the mid-inguinal point. Assess for a radio-femoral delay.
- Palpate for a *popliteal pulse* – Flex the knee and wrap both hands around knee with fingertips into the popliteal fossa and compress artery against tibia posteriorly. Note the popliteal pulse is often difficult to assess as the popliteal artery lies deep within the popliteal fossa.
- Palpate the *dorsalis pedis pulse* – Palpate between the head of the first and second metatarsals. Ask the patient to bring their big toe towards their face. The pulse is lateral to the tendon of extensor hallucis longus (EHL). Note the dorsalis pedis pulse is absent in 10% of normal individuals.
- Palpate the *posterior tibial pulse* – Posterior to the medial malleolus.

Auscultation

Upper limb

- Listen for bruits in the supraclavicular fossa, infraclavicular space (subclavian) and over the carotid artery.

Lower limb

- Listen for bruits in the abdomen (AAA, renal, iliacs) groin (femoral) and lower limb (adductor hiatus – Lies two-thirds along a line drawn from the ASIS to the adductor tubercle).

Special tests

Ankle-Brachial Pressure Index (Figure 10.2)

Record the systolic blood pressure in the upper limbs. Take the *higher* of the two readings. Locate the dorsalis pedis and posterior tibial pulses with the handheld Doppler and inflate the cuff until the Doppler sound disappears. Slowly deflate and record the pressure at which the sound reappears. Take the *higher* of the two readings (posterior tibial or dorsalis pedis). The ABPI is the ratio of the best foot systolic to brachial systolic pressure (normal > 1.0; claudication 0.4–0.7; critical ischaemia 0.1–0.4).

Allen's Test

The patient should make a fist with their hand. Now occlude both radial and ulnar arteries. When the patient opens their palm, it should be white. You may now release the pressure on the ulnar artery (the hand should re-perfuse). Repeat the test, i.e.

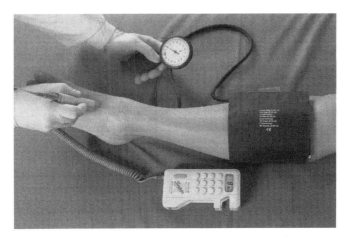

Figure 10.2 Handheld Doppler probe and sphygmomanometer used to determine systolic pressure in the dorsalis pedis artery, as part of assessing the ankle–brachial pressure index (ABPI).

make a fist, occlude both arteries, open palm and now release the radial artery. This test demonstrates collateral circulation.

Buerger's test

Elevate the patient's straight leg off the examination couch. The leg angle from the examination couch when the leg turns white is Buerger's angle (<20° = severe ischaemia). Assist the patient in allowing them to drop their leg over the side of the couch and inspect for reactive hyperaemia.

Complete the peripheral vascular examination

- Perform a full cardiovascular assessment
- Perform a full neurological examination of the upper and lower limbs
- Perform a full abdominal examination (to exclude an AAA)
- Exclude thoracic outlet obstruction (*Adson's test, Wright's manoeuvre and Roos' test*)
- Using a handheld Doppler to assess pulses and character of waveforms, i.e. normal triphasic, biphasic (moderate stenosis), monophasic (severe stenosis) or absent waveforms
- Request x-rays (chest x-ray [CXR] to identify a cervical rib) or computed tomography (CT) scan (to identify an AAA)
- Arterial duplex
- Arterial angiogram
- Assess the impact of the joint condition on the patient's life
- Assess the patient's fitness for surgery

Thank the patient and wash hands.

Summarise and offer your differential diagnosis.

VENOUS SYSTEM: EXAMINATION FOR VARICOSE VEINS

Introduction and handwash

Have the patient standing. The patient's groin and lower limbs should be fully exposed.

Ask the patient whether they have any pain.

Inspection

General

- Look around bed for walking aids and support stockings.
- Look at the patient as a whole (well/unwell; pain/pain free).

Specific

- Ask the patient to stand with one leg in front of the other. You must inspect from the front, sides and behind (Figure 10.3).
- Assess for varicose veins (abnormal prominent superficial, tortuous and dilated veins), note their distribution (long or short saphenous veins or both) and location (the medial gaiter area).
- Assess for surgical scars in the groin and lower limbs.
- Assess for saphena varix (varicosity in the saphenous vein at its confluence with the femoral vein) (Figure 10.4).

Inspect the lower limbs for '*chronic venous hypertension*':

- Ulceration
- Haemosiderin deposition
- Thrombophlebitis
- Venous eczema and stars
- Lipodermatosclerosis ('*inverted champagne bottle leg*')
- Pitting oedema
- Healed ulceration (*atrophie blanche*) (Figure 10.5) and ankle flare (*corona phlebectatica*)
- Loss of hair
- Shiny skin

Palpation (ask the patient whether they are in pain before you begin)

- Temperature of the lower limbs (with the back of the hand)
- Tenderness
- Pitting oedema
- Palpate the course of long and short saphenous veins
- Palpate for pitting oedema

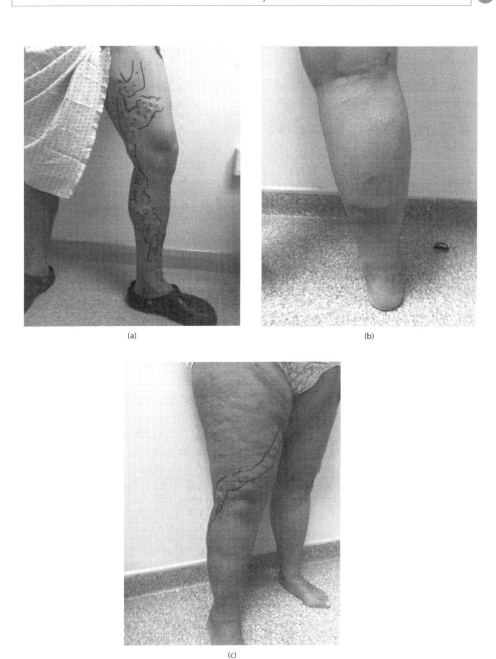

(a)

(b)

(c)

Figure 10.3 Varicose veins. (a) Left leg varicose veins in the distribution of an incompetent long saphenous vein (marked for intervention). (b) Right leg varicose veins in the distribution of the short saphenous system with a recent episode of phlebitis. (c) Varicose veins in distribution of an isolated incompetent proximal anterolateral tributary of the long saphenous system with associated gaiter area skin changes.

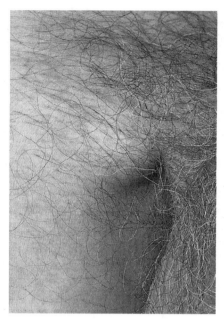

Figure 10.4 A saphena varix.

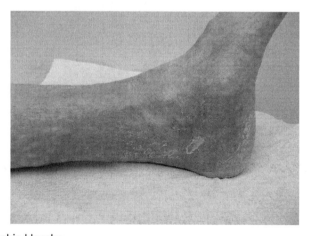

Figure 10.5 Atrophie blanche.

- Palate for the groin for regional lymph nodes
- Palpate for a saphena varix
- Perform the *cough test* to assess for a cough impulse or thrill

Identify the saphenofemoral junction (SFJ) in the groin (just medial to the femoral pulse). Whilst your index finger is over this junction, ask the patient to cough.

Percussion

- Perform the *tap test* (Chevrier's percussion test).

  - Tap proximally and palpate distally (retrograde transmission) to detect venous valvular incompetence/reflux.
  - Tap distally and palpate proximally (orthograde transmission) to assess venous continuity, venous patency and to detect thrombosis/venous occlusion.

Auscultation

- Listen for bruits (arteriovenous fistulae)

Special tests

Tourniquet Test

Also known as the *Brodie-Trendelenberg test* (if your fingers or thumb are placed over the SFJ, instead of using a tourniquet). Place the patient in a supine position then elevate the lower limb to empty the veins. Apply a tourniquet high on the upper thigh and ask the patient to stand up. If the incompetence is above the tourniquet site, the veins will be controlled and will not fill. If the incompetence is below the level of the tourniquet, the vein will fill. This should be repeated with the tourniquet positioned at a lower level on the thigh.

Perthes' Test

Place the tourniquet on the patient's thigh and then ask the patient to stand on their toes. If the veins enlarge or the patient experiences pain, the deep veins are likely to be involved.

Handheld Doppler Ultrasound

The Doppler ultrasound is used to identify the femoral artery and the SFG. Then compress the patient's calf. If there is venous incompetence at the SFJ, listen for backflow.

Complete the venous system examination

- Complete your full vascular examination with ABPI of the lower limb.
- Venous duplex of the lower limbs.
- Perform a full abdominal examination (abdominal, pelvic exam, digital rectal examination and examine the external genitalia) to exclude secondary causes of varicose veins.
- Assess the impact of the joint condition on the patient's life.
- Assess the patient's fitness for surgery.

Thank the patient and wash hands

Summarise and offer your differential diagnosis

ULCER: EXAMINATION

Introduction and handwash

Have the patient sitting. The patient's whole lower limbs should be fully exposed.

Ask the patient whether they have any pain.

You will need to ascertain the underlying aetiology of the ulcer (arterial, venous, neuropathic or mixed).

Inspection

General

- Look around bed for walking aids and dressings.
- Look at the patient as a whole (well/unwell; pain/pain free).

Specific

- Inspect between the toes, tips of toes, pressure points, heel, sole, malleoli, under the fifth metatarsal head, ball of foot.
- Inspect for amputations and gangrene.
- Inspect for surgical scars (legs and groins).
- Systematically examine the ulcer and use the mnemonic 'BEDDS.'

- *Base* – Healthy, slough, necrotic, avascular, malignant change, visible underlying structures (tendon/muscle/fascia/bone/ligaments/joints)
- *Edges* – Irregular/regular; Sloping/punched out
- *Depth* – In millimeters or superficial/full thickness down to bone/tendon/fascia/muscle)
- *Discharge* – Serous, sanguineous, serosanguinous, clear, purulent
- *Skin* – Chronic venous hypertension, other ulcers and varicose veins
- *Size* – Width by length
- *Shape* – Regularly round, irregularly round
- *Site* – Venous: medial gaiter area
- Arterial – Periphery of limbs and pressure areas
- Neuropathic – Sites of trauma and sole of foot or heel

Palpation (ask the patient whether they are in pain before you begin and you should put on gloves for this part of the examination)

- Assess for temperature (with the back of the hand)
- Assess for tenderness
- Assess for regional lymph nodes

Special tests

Ascertain the underlying aetiology of the ulcer (Figures 10.6 and 10.7)

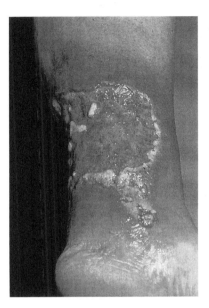

Figure 10.6 A venous ulcer.

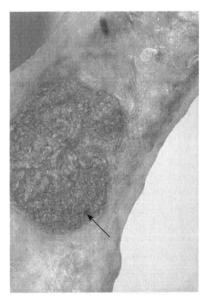

Figure 10.7 A Marjolin's ulcer (a squamous cell cancer arising in a chronic venous ulcer; arrow).

Arterial ulcers:

- Perform a full vascular examination of the lower limbs (including capillary refill time and full assessment of the distal pulses)

Neuropathic/Diabetic ulcers:

- Perform a full neurological assessment of the lower limbs
- Determine blood glucose

Venous ulcers:

- Perform a full vascular examination of the lower limbs

Complete the ulcer examination

- Complete your full vascular, venous and neurological examinations
- Blood tests to exclude infection, diabetes and hypercholesteremia
- Arterial and venous duplex
- ABPI
- Duplex scans (arterial/venous)
- Arterial angiogram

Thank the patient and wash hands.

Summarise and offer your differential diagnosis.

CHAPTER 11: PROCEDURAL SKILLS

Key Topics

Procedures

Radiology

Operations

KEY TOPICS

Informed consent

What is consent?

Informed consent is the process by which a patient is provided with sufficient information to make an informed, reasoned decision regarding the proposed treatment. In surgical practice, respect for autonomy translates into the clinical duty to obtained informed consent before the commencement of treatment.

In order for consent to be valid, three requirements must be met. It must be

- Informed
- Voluntary (non-coerced)
- Patient should be competent

Competence to take the decision requires the ability

- To understand the information given
- To retain and believe it
- To weigh up the information given to reach a reasoned decision

What types of consent do you know of?

- Implied consent (e.g. when a patient holds out their arm to have a blood test)
- Verbal consent
- Written consent

What types of consent form might you find in the hospital setting?

- Consent Form 1 – Patient agreement to investigation or treatment. Standard consent form used for adults undergoing an operation under general anaesthetic.
- Consent Form 2 – Parental agreement to investigation or treatment for a child or young person.
- Consent Form 3 – Patient/parental agreement to investigation or treatment (procedures where consciousness not impaired). In other words, procedures under local anaesthesia or sedation (e.g. endoscopy).
- Consent Form 4 – Form for adults who are unable to consent to investigation or treatment (usually patients on the intensive care unit).

What information is required for informed consent to take place?

This is easily remembered using the mnemonic **CONSENTS**:

C condition and natural history

O options/alternatives (conservative/medical/surgical)

N name of procedure

S side effects and complications

E extra procedures involved (stomas, drains, tracheostomy etc.)

N name of the person operating

T trial and training (research and medical students)

S second opinion

Finally answer any questions the patient may have about the procedure and ensure they are happy to proceed before asking them to sign the consent form.

Who provides consent in the following clinical situations?

A 15-year-old boy requires an orchidopexy.

- The parent or guardian gives consent on their behalf. The procedure and its potential risks are explained to the child and the parent or guardian.

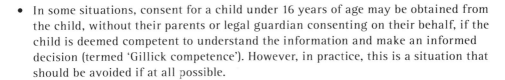

- In some situations, consent for a child under 16 years of age may be obtained from the child, without their parents or legal guardian consenting on their behalf, if the child is deemed competent to understand the information and make an informed decision (termed 'Gillick competence'). However, in practice, this is a situation that should be avoided if at all possible.

A 75-year old who in unconscious and requires an emergency operation.

- In the case of an unconscious patient, the law recognises that it is in the patient's best interest for such an emergency treatment to go ahead. However, it is always good practice to involve the next of kin in any decision. If no next of kin is available, it is wise to obtain a colleague's agreement with the surgical procedure proposed and carefully document this in the notes.

Diathermy

What is diathermy?

Diathermy (electrocoagulation) is the passage of high-frequency alternating current (AC) to produce a localised heat effect resulting in local tissue destruction, sealing of blood vessels to arrest bleeding and cutting of tissues.

What are the different types of diathermy?

- *Monopolar (Unipolar)* – The current flows from a current generator to a small active electrode held by the operating surgeon. The tip of the electrode represents a point of high current density and where the heat is generated. The current then flows through the patient and ends at a second electrode, the diathermy plate.
- *Bipolar* – The current passes down one arm of the forceps, through structures between the forceps tips and then returns through the other arm of the forceps. A loop is created (Figure 11.1).

What is the surface area of the monopolar diathermy plate?

- Surface area – ≥ 70 cm^2

What are the different diathermy modes?

- *Cutting* – In this cutting or continuous mode, an electrical arc is used to cut tissues and cauterise the divided surface. Cell water is vaporised resulting in tissue destruction.
- *Coagulation* – In this coagulation or fulguration mode, a pulsed high intensity output passes through the tissues causing tissue desiccation and sealing of blood vessels.
- *Blend* – A mixture of cutting and coagulation modes.

Can diathermy be used in patients with pacemakers?

Diathermy can interfere with pacemaker function. The two major potential complications are reprogramming and myocardial burns. This can result in cardiac arrhythmias

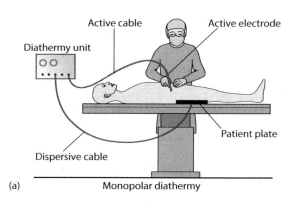

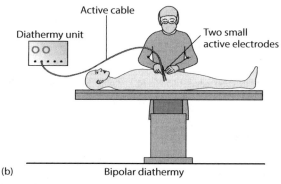

Figure 11.1 The principles of diathermy. (a) Monopolar diathermy. (b) Bipolar diathermy. (From Royal College of Surgeons of England, *The Intercollegiate Basic Surgical Skills Course Participants Handbook*, edns 1–4. London: RCS, 2007. With permission.)

or cardiac damage when diathermy is used in patients with implanted or external pacemakers. The risk is increased if the pacemaker and its connections are in the direct pathway between the active electrode and the plate. Diathermy should be avoided in patients with electronic implants. Avoid diathermy completely if possible, but if it is necessary use bipolar. If monopolar must be used, place the patient plate so that diathermy current flows well away from the pacemaker system and use only short bursts (<2 seconds) at the lowest power setting possible. External pacing should be available in case of cardiac dysfunction.

Who is responsible for the use and complications of diathermy in the operating theatre?

- The operating surgeon

What are the potential complications of diathermy?

- Burn and thermal injury are the major complications of diathermy use resulting from
  - Incorrect application of the diathermy plate
  - Patient in contact with earth metals
  - Poor technique

- Direct coupling of instruments (see Figure 11.2).
- Capacitance coupling – Inductive coupling occurs when an electrode is inside an insulator with a further conduction outside (i.e. laparoscopic ports) (see Figure 11.3).
- Arcing can occur with metal instruments and implants.
- Fire and explosions as a result of pooling of alcohol-based skin preparations (e.g. pooling in umbilicus).
- Explosions. Sparks can ignite volatile anaesthetic gases. Use of diathermy on large bowel should therefore be avoided.
- 'Channelling' effects can occur if diathermy is used on a viscus with a narrow pedicle (e.g. penis or testis).
- Carcinogenic surgical smoke.

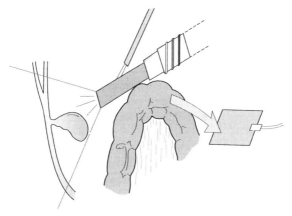

Figure 11.2 Direct coupling between bowel and laparoscope, which is touching the activated probe.

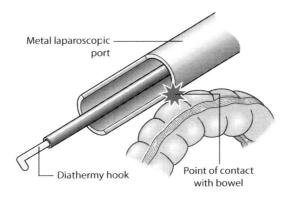

Figure 11.3 Capacitance coupling during laparoscopic surgery. (From Royal College of Surgeons of England, *The Intercollegiate Basic Surgical Skills Course Participants Handbook*, edns 1–4. London: RCS, 2007. With permission.)

How do diathermy burns occur?

- Inadequate application of the plate electrode.
- Spirit burns.
- Patient touching earthed metal, such as drip stands or the metal areas of the operating table.
- Faulty insulation of diathermy leads.
- Inadvertent activity.
  - Accidental activation of foot pedal
  - Not replacing electrode in quiver after use
  - Accidental contact of active electrode with retractors, instruments, towel clips etc.
- Use of diathermy on appendages (e.g. penis), so-called 'channelling effects'. Channelling effects occur because heat is produced where the current density is greatest.

The patient plate electrode:

- Incorrect placement is the most common cause of accidental diathermy burns.
- It requires good contact on dry, shaved skin and kinking must be avoided.
- It is normally placed on the patient's thigh.
- Contact surface area should be at least 70 cm² to minimise the risk of heating.
- It should be placed away from bony prominences and scar tissue (which have poor blood supply and therefore poor heat distribution).
- Should be placed away from metallic implants (e.g. prosthetic hips).

What precautions should the surgeon take to make sure diathermy is used safely in the operating theatre?

- Wipe excess alcoholic skin preparation to dryness.
- Consider a bipolar technique.
- Avoid high-voltage modes.
- Check the patient plate electrode is used correctly.
- Ensure the patient is not touching earthed metal.
- Avoid non-contact (open circuit) activation.
- Use only enough power to achieve the desired effect.
- Check insulation (but remember that even intact insulation may fail with high voltages due to the effects of capacitance coupling).
- Do not reuse single-use electrodes.
- Place the diathermy in a safe, insulated container (quiver) when it is not being used.
- In laparoscopic surgery, keep the active electrode in full view at all times.

Lasers in the operating theatre

What is a laser and what are its properties?

Laser stands for Light Amplification by the Stimulated Emission of Radiation

Laser emissions are

- Collimated – Parallel output beam results in little energy loss
- Coherent – Waves are all in phase resulting in little loss of energy
- Monochromic – All of the same wavelength

The effects of a laser depend on photochemical, photomechanical and photothermal factors. Tissue penetration increases with wavelength. Pulsing of output can reduce thermal damage.

How can lasers be classified?

Lasers are classified according to the amount of damage they can cause

Class 1 – Generally safe
Class 2 – Safe within the time of the blink reflex
Class 3 – Cause blindness after short exposure from mirrored surfaces
Class 4 – Unsafe even with reflection from non-mirrored surfaces

All medical lasers belong to class 4, so both patients and operators are required to wear goggles.

What are the risks associated with lasers?

Patient risks:

- Excessive burning
- Scar formation
- Visceral perforation
- Airway fire

Operator risks:

- Accidental skin exposure
- Corneal or retinal burns
- Cataracts

Environmental risk:

- Fire risk

What safety precautions should be taken when using lasers in the operating theatre?

- Dedicated laser protection advisor/officer.
- Adequate training by nominated users.
- Designated laser controlled area, with warning signs, avoiding reflective surfaces with matt-black surfaces (see Figure 11.4).
- No inflammable fixtures or furnishings in operating theatre.
- Eye protection worn by all persons in the laser controlled area at all times.
- Laser fitted with a key switch.
- Cut-out devices and shrouded foot pedals to minimise the risk of unintended operation.
- Surgeon should warn the theatre staff before firing the laser (and when not being used the laser should be remain in 'standby' mode).

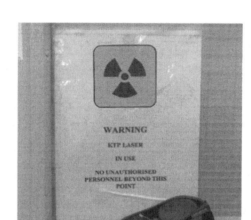

Figure 11.4 Lasers in the operating theatre.

- Care with the direction of the laser beam is critical in safe usage.
- Laser resistant endotracheal tubes (to prevent airway fires).
- Wet swabs may be used to decrease risk of inadvertent laser damage to adjacent tissues.
- Regular maintenance.
- Adequate ventilation for laser plume.

Laparoscopy and creation of a pneumoperitoneum

What are the advantages and disadvantages of minimal access surgery?

Advantages:

- Decreased wound size
- Reduced wound infection, dehiscence, bleeding, herniation and nerve entrapment
- Decrease in wound pain
- Improved mobility
- Decreased wound trauma
- Decreased heat loss
- Improved vision

Disadvantages:

- Reliance on remote vision and operating
- Loss of tactile feedback
- Dependence on hand-eye coordination
- Difficulty with haemostasis
- Reliance on new techniques
- Extraction of larger specimens

What are the complications of laparoscopy?

- Complications of trocar insertion:
  - Bleeding, damage to underlying viscera
- Complications of gas carbon dioxide insufflation. These can be classified into cardiovascular, respiratory and metabolic complications, for example:
  - Cardiovascular – Air embolism, decreased venous return and cardiac output (secondary to caval compression), cardiac dysrhythmias, decreased renal perfusion
  - Respiratory – Diaphragmatic splinting, pneumothorax, pneumomediastinum, ruptured bullae, diaphragmatic irritation (resulting in shoulder-tip pain), subcutaneous emphysema
  - Metabolic – Acidosis (metabolic or respiratory), increased risk of DVTs (venous pooling), aspiration (from increased intraabdominal pressure)
- Complications of diathermy:
  - Direct coupling (instrument to instrument coupling), capacitance coupling, insulation defects, inappropriate or inadvertent activation of electrodes out of view, gas explosions, burning the wrong structure, retained heat
- Complications of portal sites:
  - Bleeding, infection, port site hernias

What is capacitance coupling?

Also known as 'inductive coupling', a capacitor is effectively created by having an insulator sandwiched between two electrodes, with high-frequency AC passing through. This can occur by having the core of the diathermy hook acting as one electrode and the metal laparoscopic port acting as another electrode with a layer of insulation in between. Current flowing through the active diathermy hook can induce current in the metal port, which can potentially damage adjacent tissues. Fortunately such incidents are rare and can be prevented by using non-conducting ports (Figure 11.5).

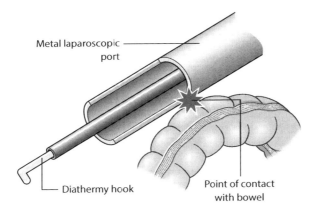

Metal laparoscopic port

Diathermy hook

Point of contact with bowel

Figure 11.5 Capacitance coupling during laparoscopic surgery. (From Royal College of Surgeons of England, *The Intercollegiate Basic Surgical Skills Course Participants Handbook*, edns 1–4. London: RCS, 2007. With permission.)

Local anaesthetics

What are the maximum safe doses for local anaesthetics?

- Lignocaine 3 mg/kg (7 mg/kg with adrenaline)
- Bupivacaine 2 mg/kg
- Prilocaine 6 mg/kg (9 mg/kg with adrenaline)
- Ropivacaine 3–4 mg/kg
- Levobupivacaine 2 mg/kg

What is the difference between lignocaine and bupivacaine?

Lignocaine – Early onset of action (2–3 minutes), short acting (1–2 hours), good sensory block

Bupivacaine – Slower onset of action (10–15 minutes), long lasting (4–6 hours), more cardiotoxic

What are the benefits and risks of using adrenaline in local anaesthetics?

Benefits:

- Less bleeding (vasoconstriction)
- Prolonged duration of action
- Higher doses can be used
- Reduced systemic absorption and decreased risk of toxicity

Risks:

- Increased risk of ischaemic necrosis when operating on appendages supplied by end arteries (digits, penis etc.).
- Increased risk of cardiac dysrhythmias.
- It can precipitate critical ischaemia in poorly vascularised tissue.
- Reactive hyperaemia can occur in the post-operative period with increased risk of bleeding and haematoma.

What is the local anaesthetic of choice when performing a Bier's block and why?

Prilocaine. Intravenous (IV) regional anaesthesia under tourniquet control is a simple method of producing short-term anaesthesia of the distal arm or leg, first described by August Bier in 1908. The drug of choice is prilocaine because it is the least cardiotoxic and has the largest therapeutic index.

What are the signs of local anaesthesia toxicity and how would you manage it?

Local anaesthetic toxicity principally results in effects on the central nervous system and cardiovascular system. One of the earliest and reliable signs of systemic toxicity is perioral paraesthesia. Other early symptoms include tinnitus and visual disturbances. These are followed by dizziness, which may progress to convulsions, cardiac arrhythmias, collapse and even death.

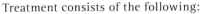

Treatment consists of the following:

- Informing the crash team, anaesthetist and/or Intensive Therapy Unit (ITU).
- Supportive management with 100% oxygen, IV access, fluids etc.
- Maintaining the airway (by intubation if necessary).
- Establishing an electrocardiogram (ECG) monitor as cardiac arrhythmias can occur.
- Cardiopulmonary resuscitation and/or inotropic support if required.
- Controlling convulsions with IV benzodiazepines and/or phenytoin.
- Increasing evidence suggests that IV infusion of lipid emulsions can reverse the cardiac and neurologic effects of local-anaesthetic toxicity and guidelines for its use exist in most anaesthetic units.

Case Study

You plan to excise a lipoma in an 85-year-old gentleman under local anaesthesia, since he is otherwise unfit for a general anaesthetic. He weighs 60 kg. How much 1% plain lignocaine can be used safely?

- The maximum safe dose of plain lignocaine = 3 mg/kg × 60 kg = 180 mg.
- As a rule, when converting % to mg/mL always multiply by a factor of 10.
- Therefore 1% lignocaine = 10 mg/mL.
- 180 mg lignocaine is equivalent to 180 mg ÷ 10 mg/mL = 18 mL of 1% lignocaine.
- Therefore up to 18 mL of 1% plain lignocaine may be given safely.

If you use the maximum dose of lignocaine, can you still infiltrate the wound with bupivacaine at the end of the operation to achieve longer lasting analgesia?

Both lignocaine and bupivacaine have maximum safe doses of 2–3 mg/kg. The important point here is that the effects are additive, so one cannot simply switch agents when the maximum safe dose is approaching. Similarly, mixing the two agents together (to provide both a rapid onset and long duration of action) does not allow an increased dose.

Sutures

The examiner may ask you to demonstrate your surgical sills in suturing. Practice your technique on models and patients prior to the examination.

What is a suture?

A suture is a material used to tie or approximate tissues together.

In addition, a suture is a joint with minimal connective tissue located in the skull vault (e.g. coronal and sagittal sutures).

What are the different types of sutures?

Sutures are classified as follows:

Absorbable or non-absorbable, natural or synthetic and monofilament or braided. Sutures may also be classified by size (e.g. 5/0, 4/0, 3/0 etc.)

- Absorbable – PDS (polydioxanone), vicryl (polyglactin) and monocryl
- Non-absorbable – Steel, prolene (polypropylene), nylon (ethilon) and silk
- Natural – Silk and catgut
- Synthetic – Vicryl and PDS
- Monofilament – PDS and prolene
- Polyfilament/braided – Vicryl and silk

How are sutures broken down?

Sutures are broken down by

- Proteolytic digestion (e.g. catgut)
- Hydrolysis (e.g. vicryl)

What makes a good suture material?

An ideal suture is

- All purpose, i.e. can be used for all types of surgery
- Easy to handle
- Predictable behaviour in tissues
- Maintains adequate tensile strength
- Minimal tissue reaction
- Holds securely
- No memory
- Inexpensive
- Easily sterilised
- Predictable performance
- Has high breaking strength
- Inert (non-electrolytic, non-shrinkage, non-capillary, non-allergenic and non-carcinogenic)

What type of suture is vicryl?

Vicryl (polyglactin) is an absorbable, synthetic, braided polymeric suture. It produces a minimal tissue reaction. It is absorbed between 56 and 70 days and provides adequate support for around 30 days.

What type of suture is silk?

Silk is a non-absorbable, natural, braided suture. It is biodegradable. Its tensile strength lasts up to 1 year. It causes an inflammatory tissue reaction and should be avoided in the placement of vascular prostheses or artificial heart valves.

Needles

What are the different parts of a needle?

A needle is comprised of a point, body and swage (Figure 11.6).

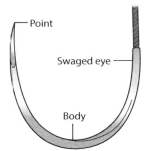

Figure 11.6 The basic parts of a needle. (From Royal College of Surgeons of England, *The Intercollegiate Basic Surgical Skills Course Participants Handbook,* edns 1–4. London: RCS, 2007. With permission.)

How are needles classified?

Needles can be classified by shape, type and effect (Figure 11.7).

Shape:

- Straight
- Curved
  - 1/4 circle
  - 3/8 circle
  - 1/2 circle
  - 5/8 circle
- J shaped
- Compound curve

Type:

- *Round-bodied needles* – They are designed to separate *(not cut)* tissue fibres. They may be used in soft tissues. After the needle is passed, the tissue closes tightly around the suture material to form a leak-proof line.

  - Intestinal
  - Heavy
  - Blunt taper point
  - Blunt point

- *Cutting needles* – They are designed for tough or dense tissues.

  - Tapercut
  - Conventional cutting
  - Reverse cutting

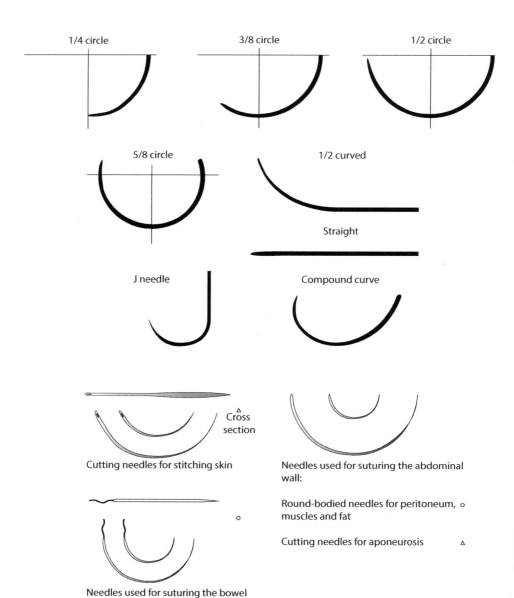

Figure 11.7 Types of needle.

Effect:

- *Traumatic needles* – Needles with holes or eyes. They are supplied separate from the suture thread. The suture is threaded on-site. A needle with an eye carries a double strand, which creates a larger hole and disruption to the underlying tissue. These are rarely seen nowadays but are occasionally still used, e.g. aneurysm needle.

- *Atraumatic needles* – This eyeless needle is swaged (pre-mounted) to a suture. This reduces handling, preparation time and causes less trauma to the underlying tissues.

What advantage does a reverse cutting needle have over a cutting needle?

In a reverse cutting needle, the cutting edge is situated on the outside of the needle and is therefore less likely to cut through the tissues. In addition, by having the apex cutting edge on the outside of the needle curvature, this improves the strength of the needle and increases its resistance to bending. Reverse cutting needles, however, do require more force to penetrate the tissue.

How are surgical needles chosen?

Remember the mnemonic PATS

- P Procedure
- A Access
- T Tissue
- S Surgeons preference

PROCEDURES

Urinary catheterisation

Introduction, explain the procedure, confirm indication for catheterisation and obtain informed consent.

Positioning

- For female patients, request a chaperone.
- The patient is in a supine position. In males, the legs should be extended.
- In females, the knees should be bent with the heels together and the thighs abducted.

Preparation of equipment

- Wash your hands.
- Position yourself with your back to the patient and place the trolley in front of you.
- Open the non-sterile outer packaging of the catharisation pack and slide the sterile pack on to the procedure trolley.
- While maintaining asepsis, open the catharisation pack and create a sterile field. Pour sterile chlorhexidine solution into a galley pot and open the following items on to the sterile field:
  - Lignocaine gel a 10-mL syringe to inflate the catheter balloon
  - A Foley catheter (the smallest practicable urinary catheter is used, typically 12-gauge in females and 14-gauge in males)

Procedure

- Put on sterile gloves.
- Place the sterile drapes (found in the pack) around the patient's perineum and thighs to create a sterile field.
- For male patients, using your gloved hand closest to the patient (and/or a swab), retract the foreskin and hold the penis until the procedure is complete. In the case of female patients, this hand should be used to hold the labia apart.
- The 'holding' hand should not touch the catheter.
- For male patients, the 'clean' gloved hand should then be used to clean the glans penis with cotton swabs soaked in chlorhexidine solution. In female patients, the urethral meatus should be cleaned from the pubis towards the anus to avoid contamination from the perineum.
- Holding the penis perpendicular to the body, the 'clean' hand should then introduce the nozzle of the lignocaine lubricating gel into the urethral meatus and insert approximately 30–50 mL of gel into the urethra.
- Ideally, wait for 5 minutes for the local anaesthetic to take effect.
- A sterile receiver containing the catheter should then be placed between the patient's legs, and the 'clean' hand should be used to insert the catheter.
- The catheter should be gently advanced to the hilt.
- When urine is seen to flow, the balloon should be gently inflated with 5–10 mL of sterile water, after which the catheter should be slowly withdrawn so that the balloon rests at the bladder neck.
- Send the urine sample for microscopy, culture and sensitivities (MC&S).
- The catheter should then be attached to a drainage system (e.g. leg bag, urometer or drainage bag) and secured.
- Replace the foreskin.

Complications of urinary catheterisation

Immediate complications:

- Failure to catheterise
- Bleeding
- Urethral and prostatic trauma

Early complications:

- Infection
- Blockage
- Paraphimosis

Late complications:

- False passage
- Long-term catheter

Central line insertion

Introduction, explain the procedure, confirm indication for central line insertion and obtain informed consent

Positioning (for right internal jugular [RIJ] vein catheterisation)

- Place the patient in a supine position in reverse Trendelenburg position to engorge the neck veins and to prevent air embolism.
- Tilt the patient's head to the left side.

Preparation

- Wash your hands and put on a pair of sterile gloves.
- Gather the following equipment on a procedure trolley:
  - Sterile dressing pack
  - Gown and sterile gloves
  - Betadine
  - Lignocaine
  - Central line
  - Normal saline flush
  - Guidewire
  - Vessel dilator
  - Introducer needle
  - 1/0 silk suture plus adhesive dressing

Procedure

- Scrub up, gown and glove.
- Prepare the right side of the patient's neck with betadine and create a sterile field around the puncture site using the sterile drapes within the dressing pack.
- Flush each central line lumen with normal saline.
- Palpate for the carotid artery with the left hand and using the right hand infiltrate the skin lateral to the artery and between the heads of sternocleidomastoid with 1% lignocaine using a 23-gauge needle.
- Change to a larger 21-gauge needle. Angle the needle at 45° to the skin and aiming towards the ipsilateral nipple, aspirate and infiltrate the subcutaneous tissues with local anaesthetic and locate the RIJ vein.
- When a flashback is seen, withdraw the needle and advance the larger bore introducer needle (attached to a syringe) in the line of the previous needle and locate the RIJ vein.

- Once the vein has been punctured and dark non-pulsatile venous blood can be freely aspirated, detach the syringe from the needle and feed the guidewire through the lumen of the needle. There should be no resistance.
- Once approximately half the length of the guidewire has been inserted, remove the needle.
- Nick the skin at the puncture site with the scalpel provided and thread the dilator over the guidewire to the hilt.
- Remove the dilator and feed the catheter over the guidewire. Once the central venous catheter is in place, remove the guidewire.
- Check that blood can be aspirated from each of the lumens and flush each lumen with normal saline.
- Secure the central line in place using 1/0 silk and apply an adhesive dressing.
- Dispose of the clinical waste and sharps appropriately.

Closure

Explain to the patient that the central line has been successfully inserted and that a chest radiograph will need to be performed (to exclude a pneumothorax) prior to its use.

Complications of central venous line insertion:

- Pneumothorax
- Haemothorax
- Bleeding with or without haematoma
- Thrombosis of vein
- Inadvertent arterial cannulation
- Catheter tip embolus
- Air embolus
- Arrhythmias
- Infection

Arterial blood–gas sampling

Introduction, explain the procedure, confirm indication and obtain informed consent.

Positioning the patient

- Wash your hands or use alcohol gel.
- Ensure that the patient is seated or lying comfortably.
- Select the artery to be used, in the following order of preference – Radial, femoral and brachial artery.
- If the radial artery is selected, an Allen test should be performed prior to arterial sampling to ensure that the collateral blood supply to the hand from the ulnar artery is intact. Support the wrist on a pillow.

Preparation

- Wash your hands and put on a pair of gloves.
- Gather the following equipment:
  - Heparinised syringe
  - 23–25 gauge needle
  - Alcohol swab

Procedure

- Clean the arterial puncture site with an alcohol swab.
- Wait 30 seconds for the alcohol to evaporate.
- Hyperextend the wrist joint (helping to bring the artery to the surface) and palpate the radial artery proximally and distally, using the index and middle finger.
- Expel the heparin from the syringe completely and, holding the syringe like a pencil with the bevel pointed upwards, enter the skin at an angle of 60°–90° between the two fingers.
- Advance the needle, maintaining a slight negative pressure until a bright red flashback is seen. Some syringes fill spontaneously due to the pressure in the artery, while others require gentle aspiration.
- When 1–2 mL of blood has been obtained, withdraw the needle and apply pressure to the puncture site for 5 minutes or longer if the patient is on anticoagulation.
- Expel any air within the syringe. Remove the needle into a sharps container and cap the syringe.
- Analyse the blood sample obtained (Figure 11.8).

Joint aspiration

Introduction, explain the procedure, confirm indication and obtain informed consent.

Positioning the patient

- Wash your hands and put on a pair of gloves.
- Ensure that the patient is comfortable in a supine position with the knee fully extended and exposed.
- Identify the optimal site of aspiration – The medial aspect of the patella in the patellar-femoral groove of the left knee.

Preparation

Gather the following equipment:

- Lignocaine 2%
- Betadine
- Dressing pack
- Specimen pot
- Syringe

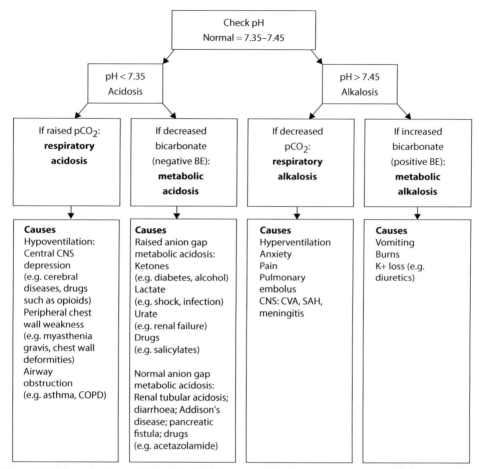

Figure 11.8 Normal values: pCO2 = 4.3–6.0 kPa; plasma bicarbonate = 22–26 mmol/L; base excess (BE) ±2.

- 25-gauge and 21-gauge needles
- Glucose tube

Using a procedure trolley, open out a sterile dressing pack to create a sterile field.

The dressing pack should contain a waste disposal bag. Attach this to the side of the procedure trolley for convenience and, while maintaining the sterile field, open all equipment.

Procedure

- Scrub up, gown and glove.
- Clean the left knee with Betadine and, using the drapes within the dressing pack, create a sterile field around the marked puncture site.

- Allow the Betadine to dry, and clean the puncture site with an alcohol swab (as Betadine can invalidate culture results).
- Anaesthetise the skin at the puncture site with lignocaine (2%), raising a bleb with a 25-gauge needle (note that lignocaine is bactericidal). Wait for the anaesthetic to take effect.
- Insert the needle through the skin and into the knee joint, aspirating as you advance the needle. Stop when fluid is encountered.
- Withdraw as much of the fluid as possible and fill the two specimen pots and the glucose tube.
- Withdraw the needle and apply pressure.
- Dispose of the waste and needles appropriately.

Surgical scrubbing, gowning and gloving
Preparation

- Remove watch and hand jewellery, including rings.
- Nails should be short and clean (with no nail varnish).
- Surgical scrubs (greens), shoes/clogs and disposable cap must be worn in the operating room. Apply a facemask before scrubbing.
- Open out a sterile gown pack. Open the outer pack consisting of a sterile pair of gloves, dropping the sterile inner gloves into the sterile field created by opening out the gown pack.

Procedure

- The first scrub of the day should last 5 minutes and subsequent scrubs should last 3 minutes.
- Turn on the water and adjust the temperature.
- Open a sterile sponge/brush pack. Note that the sponge may or may not be impregnated with surgical scrub (e.g. Betadine), and leave to one side.
- Keep your hands above your elbows and do not touch any non-sterile objects/ surfaces.
- Hold your body away from your arms.
- Wet your forearms and hands, allowing the water to drain downwards from your hands to your elbows. Do not shake your hands or arms, but allow the water to drip away.
- Using your elbow, dispense Betadine or chlorhexidine scrub. Lather the detergent and perform a pre-scrub, washing from the hands to 2 cm above the elbow and then rinsing.
- Scrub one arm completely as described below before proceeding to the other arm.
- Using the brush and nail file, brush and file under the fingernails for 30 seconds per hand.

- Scrub each of the four surfaces of each finger, the palm, the back as well as the heel of the hand for a further minute per hand.
- Discard the sponge.
- Wash from the hands to the elbows for 1 minute without retracing your steps and then rinse, allowing the water to run away from your hands to your elbow.
- Pick up the towel, ensuring that it does not make contact with either your body or any non-sterile surface, and step away from the gowning table.
- Continue to hold your hands above your elbows, and dry your hands and forearms from distal to proximal using opposite sides of the same towel for each hand and forearm. Discard the towel on completion.
- Pick up your gown with one hand. Hold the gown away from you at the neck and at chest level and allow it to unfold.
- Slip your arms into the sleeves of the gown and advance your fingertips as far as but not beyond the proximal border of the gown cuffs.
- Ask a colleague to fasten the ties at the back of the gown.
- Open out the inner glove package.
- Pick up the left glove with your sleeve-covered left hand and place it on the opposite sleeve gown with the palm of the glove facing down and the fingers pointing towards you.
- Taking the folded edge of the glove with the thumb and index finger of your sleeve-covered left hand (palm facing upwards), use your sleeve-covered right hand to stretch the glove over the sleeve-covered left hand by grasping on the outer edge of the glove fold.
- Pull any excess sleeve from inside the glove using your sleeve-covered right hand.
- Pick up the right glove under its fold with your gloved left hand and pull the glove over your right hand.
- As before, draw any excess sleeve from the gown cuffs using your left hand.
- This is the closed technique for gloving and gowning.
- Finally, take the paper belt tab found at the front of the gown and pass it to the scrub nurse/assistant.
- The assistant will take the paper tab and move behind you to pass the belt (but not the paper tab) back to you.
- Tie the belt at the front to complete gowning (Figure 11.9).

Suturing a wound

Introduction, explain the procedure, confirm indication and obtain informed consent.

Position the patient with the wound exposed.

Preparation of equipment

Wash your hands and put on a pair of gloves. Prepare the following on a procedure trolley:

- Appropriate local anaesthetic
- 10-mL syringe and 25-gauge needle

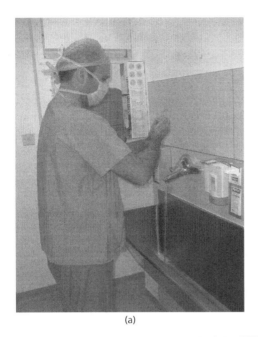

(a)

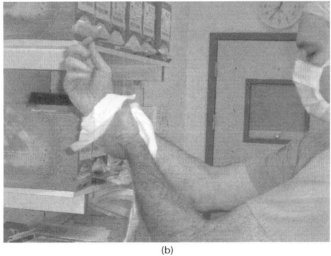

(b)

Figure 11.9 (a) and (b) Scrubbing up.

- Dressing pack
- Betadine
- Appropriate suture material and needle
- Local anaesthetics and suturing

Maximum safe dose varies with anaesthetic used and patient's weight – lignocaine (Xylocaine) safe dose: 5 mg/kg lignocaine plus adrenaline: 7 mg/kg bupivacaine (Marcain): 3 mg/kg.

Concentration in mg can be calculated by multiplying percentage concentration by 10 (e.g. 1% lignocaine contains 10 mg/mL)

Procedure

- Scrub up, gown and glove.
- Clean the wound with Betadine, starting at the centre and working outwards without retracing old ground.
- Infiltrate the wound with local anaesthetic using a 25-gauge needle, not exceeding the maximum safe amount.
- Aspirate before injecting to avoid inadvertent intra-arterial injection. (Do not use adrenaline in digits, as its peripheral vasoconstriction effect can cause ischaemia.)
- Select the appropriate suture and needle.
- Hold the forceps between thumb and index finger and use it to manipulate (not to crush) the skin edges. Forceps may be toothed (used for skin and tough tissue) or non-toothed (used for bowel and blood vessels).
- Hold the needle holder with the thumb and index fingers inserted in the bows advanced no further than the distal phalanx. Extend the index finger to steady the scissors over its joint.
- Mount the needle two-thirds of the way from its tip.
- Insert the needle at right angles to the skin, advance the needle through one skin edge, pick the needle up using forceps (not hands), remount and advance the needle through the opposite skin edge. (The distance from the skin edge should be roughly equal to the thickness of the wound for each stitch.)
- Pull the suture through, leaving the non-needle end short.
- Either instrument or hand-tie the suture, forming a reef knot, ensuring that the skin edges are 'approximated not strangulated' (Figure 11.10a).
- Hold the scissors in a similar manner to the needle holder and cut using the tips of the scissors. Use the index finger of the opposite hand to support the scissors underneath while cutting.
- Successive sutures should be equidistant at a distance of twice the wound depth (Figure 11.10b).
- The resulting closure should be 'tension free'.
- Apply the dressing.
- Dispose of sharps and clinical waste appropriately.

Closure

- Ensure that the patient is comfortable.
- Advise the patient about:
- What has been done?
- The type of suture used (i.e. 6/0 or 5/0 for face and dorsum hands; 3/0 or 4/0 for limbs)

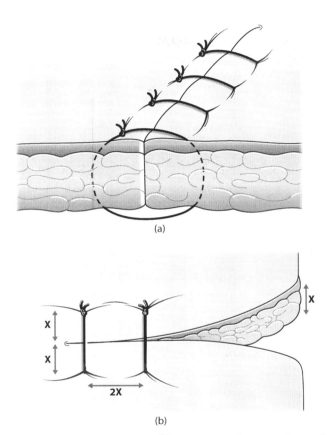

(a)

(b)

Figure 11.10 (a) Interrupted suture technique. (b) The siting of sutures. As a rule of thumb, the distance of insertion from the edge of the wound should correspond to the thickness of the tissue being sutured (x). Each successive suture should be placed at twice this distance apart (2x). (From Royal College of Surgeons of England, *The Intercollegiate Basic Surgical Skills Course Participants Handbook*, edns 1–4. London: RCS, 2007. With permission.)

- Whether the sutures need to be removed and when (i.e. skin and face on days 3–5; chest and abdomen on day 10; scalp on days 5–7)
- Dressing care
- Follow-up

Chest drain

What are the indications for chest drain insertion?

These can be divided into:

- Emergency situations – Tension pneumothorax, haemothorax, chylothorax
- Elective situations – Pleural effusion, post-operative, empyema, prophylaxis

Or classified by aetiology:

- Pneumothorax – Trauma, bullae rupture in chronic obstructive pulmonary disease [COPD], iatrogenic, spontaneous, tension
- Haemothorax – Trauma and post-operative
- Chylothorax – Post-operative, injury to thoracic duct
- Massive effusion
- Empyema
- Prophylactic – Cardiac, oesophageal or spinal surgery

Explain how you would insert a chest drain?

Introduction, explain the procedure, confirm indication and obtain informed consent

Preparation

Position

- Place the patient in either a sitting or supine position (if the cervical spine has not been cleared) with their arm, on the side that the chest drain will be placed, behind the head.
- Identify the fifth intercostal space in the mid-axillary line and mark it
- Gather the following equipment:
  - Trocar-mounted chest drain (20–36 French)
  - 1% lignocaine plus syringe and 26-gauge needle
  - Minor procedures tray
  - Betadine
  - 0 silk suture
  - Underwater seal drainage system

Procedure

- Aseptic technique should be observed.
- Scrub up and gown.
- Prepare the chest drain insertion site with Betadine and drape the patient to create a sterile field.
- Infiltrate the skin and tissues down to the pleura with local anaesthetic (always drawing back on the syringe before injecting, to avoid injecting into blood vessels).
- Wait a few minutes for the anaesthetic to take effect.
- Make a 2-cm transverse incision over the upper border of the sixth rib to avoid the neurovascular bundle.
- Bluntly dissect the subcutaneous tissue and puncture the parietal pleura using either the tip of a clamp or a gloved finger.
- Layers that must be breached (superficial to deep) = skin, subcutaneous tissue, intercostal muscles, parietal pleura to enter the pleural cavity.
- Remove the chest drain trocar.

- Clamp the proximal end of the thoracostomy to help guide the drain into position, and introduce the drain, aiming for the apex (pneumothorax) or base (haemothorax) of the lungs.
- Attach the end of the chest drain to an underwater seal system and observe for bubbling (Figure 11.12).
- Using the 0 silk suture, tie the chest tube in place using a purse-string suture.
- Apply an airtight dressing and secure the tube to the patient's chest with tape (Sleek).
- Take a chest radiograph to confirm the position of the drain.

What is the 'triangle of safety'?

This is the recommended site for insertion of a chest drain and is a triangle created by

- Mid-axillary line/anterior border of latissimus dorsi
- Lateral border of pectoralis major
- Imaginary horizontal line from the nipple
- Apex of the axilla (Figure 11.11)

What are the complications of chest drain insertion?

- Pain
- Bleeding (with or without haemothorax)
- Inadvertent puncture of lungs, heart, great vessels or abdominal organs
- Damage to surrounding structures – Neurovascular bubble under each rib, long thoracic nerve of Bell
- Damage to the intercostal vein, artery and nerve
- Infection
- Subcutaneous emphysema
- Blockage of tube
- Recurrence of pneumothorax

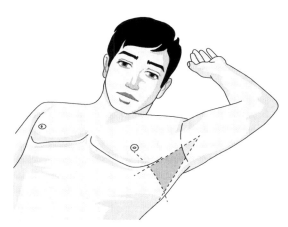

Figure 11.11 Safe triangle. (From Havelock, T, Teoh, R, Laws, D et al., *Thorax*. 65 (Suppl 2): 61–76, 2010.)

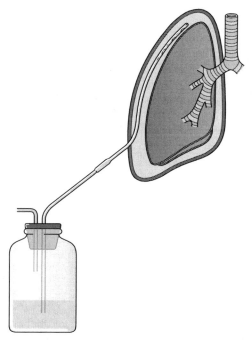

Figure 11.12 Underwater seal chest drain. (From Thomas WEG. Basic principles. In: Kingsnorth A, Majid A (eds). *Principles of Surgical Practice*, London: Greenwich Medical, 2001. With permission.)

- Persistent pneumothorax
- Failure of lung to expand (may require bronchoscopy)

Lumbar puncture

Introduction, explain the procedure, confirm indication and obtain informed consent.

Preparation

- Gather the following on the procedure trolley:
  - Spinal needles (21 gauge and 23 gauge)
  - Procedure pack (containing gallipot, gauze, sterile drapes)
  - Antiseptic Betadine/chlorhexidine solution
  - Sterile gloves and gown
  - 2% lignocaine (local anaesthetic)
  - Syringe
  - Manometer

Positioning the patient

Help to place the patient in the lateral decubitus position with the spine parallel to and at the edge of the bed. Ask the patient to draw their knees up to their stomach and flex their head to their chest, thereby flexing the vertebral column and widening the intervertebral spaces.

Procedure

Locate the L3–L4 interspace which is found along the supracristal line (an imaginary line between the iliac crests) and mark the puncture site.

The procedure should be performed using aseptic techniques.

- Open the procedure pack and prepare and check the equipment.
  - The spinal cord terminates at L1–L2 in adults and at L2–L3 in children.
  - Lumbar puncture should be performed in the L3–L4 or L4–L5 interspace.
  - L4–L5 is found along the supracristal line.
- Scrub and gown.
- Prepare (prep) the skin over the puncture site and overlying several intervertebral spaces with Betadine/chlorhexidine solution applied in a circular fashion from the centre to the periphery.
- Drape the patient.
- Using 2% lignocaine with a 25-gauge needle, raise a wheal over the puncture site to anaesthetise the skin, and then use a 21-gauge needle to infiltrate into the interspinous ligament.
- Wait a few minutes for the local anaesthetic to take effect.
- Holding the spinal needle in the index and middle finger, with the thumb holding the stylet in place, direct the needle between the spinous processes, aiming towards the umbilicus.
- Advance the needle through the skin, supraspinous ligament, interspinous ligament and ligamentum flavum, epidural space, dura and subarachnoid membrane into the subarachnoid space.
- A 'give' is felt on puncturing the ligamentum flavum, and a loss of resistance is felt as the dura is penetrated.
- Withdraw the stylet periodically to check for cerebrospinal fluid (CSF) return. If no CSF is seen, continue to advance the needle a few millimetres.
- Once a CSF flashback is seen, remove the stylet, attach the manometer and measure the pressure. Normal opening pressure is in the range 80–180 mmHg.
- Finally, collect up to 2 mL of CSF into three specimen bottles (one for biochemistry, the second for bacteriology and the third for cytology).
- Withdraw the needle and apply a dry sterile dressing.
- Dispose of the waste and sharps appropriately.

Closure

- Ask the patient to lie flat and drink plenty of fluid to reduce the risk of post-lumbar-puncture headache.
- Fill out the appropriate forms, label the specimens and dispatch them. Write a procedure note.

Differential diagnosis of CSF

Pathology	Appearance	Opening pressure	Protein (g/L)	Glucose (mg/mL)	Lymphocytes (mm⁻³)	PMNs (mm⁻³)
Normal	Clear	70–180	0.2–0.4	>50% (serum)	<5	Nil
Viral	Clear/turbid	Normal/↑	Normal/↑	>50% (serum)	10^{100}	Nil
Bacterial	Turbid/ purulent	↑	0.5–2	<50% (serum)	<50	200– 3000
Myco- bacteria	Turbid/ viscous	↑	<500	<1/3 (serum)	100–300	0–200

PMNs, polymorphonuclear neutrophils.

What are the main contraindications to lumbar puncture?

- Raised intracranial pressure
- Bleeding diathesis
- Infection
- Cardiorespiratory compromise

RADIOLOGY

Chest radiograph

General approach

Name, age and date of radiograph

Quality of the radiograph

- Rotation – Identify the medial ends of the clavicles and select one of the vertebral spinous processes that fall between them. The medial ends should be equal distant from the spinous process.
- Penetration – Look at the lower part of the cardiac shadow. The vertebral bodies should be just visible through the cardiac shadow.
- Degree of inspiration – Count the number of ribs above the diaphragm. The midpoint of the right hemidiaphragm should be between the fifth and seventh ribs anteriorly.

Orientation (PA, AP or lateral)

Look for the radiographer's marking (left or right).

Trachea

Ensure that the trachea is central. A shift may represent mediastinal or lung pathology.

Mediastinum

Check for a clear edge.

If the mediastinal diameter is more than 30% of the intrathoracic diameter, the mediastinum is enlarged.

Causes include:

- Aortic dissection
- Lymph nodes
- Thymus
- Thyroid
- Tumour

Heart

The cardiothoracic ratio is the ratio of the heart width to the chest width. It should be less than 50% (Figure 11.13).

Lung hilum

- Composed of pulmonary arteries and veins, lymph nodes and airways
- Compare shape and density
- The left hilum is higher than the right (by 1 cm)
- Describe hilar abnormalities

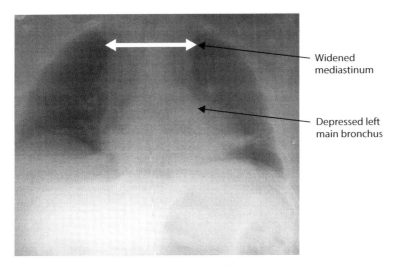

Widened mediastinum

Depressed left main bronchus

Figure 11.13 Chest radiograph showing a widened mediastinum.

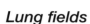

Lung fields

- These should be of equal transradiancy.
- Identify the horizontal fissure and check its position.
- Identify the costophrenic angles and ensure that they are well defined.
- Identify discrete or generalised shadows.

Increased translucency may indicate:

- Pneumothorax
- Bullous change
- Hyperinflation in chronic obstructive pulmonary disease
- Pulmonary hypertension
- Pulmonary embolism

Abnormal opacities may indicate:

- Consolidation
- Collapse
- Coin lesion, ring, shadows, linear opacities or diffuse shadows

Diaphragm

- Expansion – 6±1 anterior ribs or 9±1 posterior ribs.
- The right hemidiaphragm should be higher than the left by 3 cm.

Soft tissues

These include:

- Breast shadow
- Subcutaneous fat distribution
- Look for enlargement

Bones

- Look at the ribs, scapula and vertebrae
- Look for fractures

Summary and diagnosis

Summarise findings and formulate a differential diagnosis.

Abdominal radiograph

General approach

Name, age, date of radiograph and orientation

Quality of the radiograph

Orientation (erect or supine)
Note if contrast is present

Bones of spine and pelvis

Look for moderate degenerative change in lumbar spine or in hips, metastases or collapse.

Calcification in abdomen and pelvis

Arteries (look for a calcified abdominal aortic aneurysm or iliac arteries), lymph nodes, phleboliths and stones.

Soft tissue

Look for psoas line and kidney size and shape.

Bowel and gas pattern

Look for small bowel (central position, valvulae conniventes) or large bowel (more peripheral, haustra) obstruction and gas distribution (air in liver, biliary, genitourinary [GU], peritoneum and colonic wall) (Figure 11.14).

Summary and diagnosis

Summarise findings and formulate a differential diagnosis.

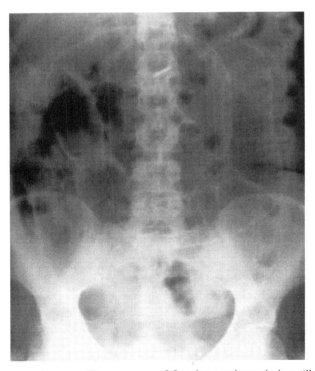

Figure 11.14 Pneumoperitoneum. The presence of free intraperitoneal air outlines the bowel so that both sides of the bowel wall can be seen (Rigler's sign).

Orthopaedic radiograph

General approach

Name, age, date of radiograph and orientation

Quality of the radiograph

Orientation

Comment on the orientation of the film, e.g. antero-posterior, lateral, etc.

Bone quality

Density and thickness

Bone alignment – Dislocations, subluxations or fractures, or deformity (Figure 11.15)

Summary and diagnosis

Summarise findings and formulate a differential diagnosis.

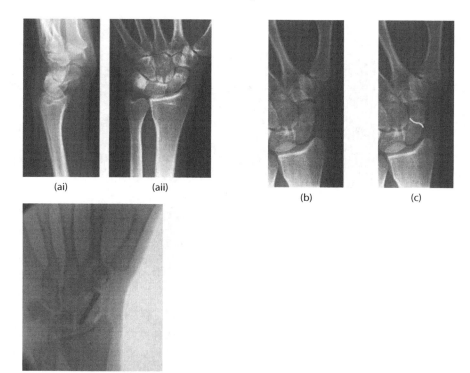

Figure 11.15 Scaphoid fracture. (a) Anteroposterior and lateral views in which the injury is difficult to see. (b, c) Oblique views with the fracture line highlighted. (d) In this case of a young patient, the fracture was treated with early fixation.

OPERATIONS

Carpal tunnel decompression

How would you perform a carpal tunnel decompression?

Can be performed:
• Under general, regional or local anaesthesia • Open or endoscopic • With or without a tourniquet

Ensure you are performing the correct operation for the correct reasons (re-take history, re-examine the patient and confirm the nerve conduction studies (electrophysiology).

- Obtain informed consent and mark the correct side.
- World Health Organisation (WHO) checklist.
- Position the arm extended and fully supinated on an arm board, with the hand held flat by a 'lead hand' retractor.
- Standard preparation and drape to expose the whole hand.
- Incision in line with third web space distal to distal wrist crease.
- Extend the incision proximal to the line of first web space (thenar eminence).
- Ensure skin incision is perpendicular to the skin.
- Protect the nerve with a Macdonald's elevator.
- Check flexor retinaculum is fully released (proximally and distally).
- Irrigation and haemostasis.
- Closure 3.0 nylon interrupted vertical mattress sutures.
- Mepore dressing and soft, non-constrictive hand bandage.
- Encourage elevation of the hand and early mobilisation.
- Prescribe analgesia.

What are the contents of the carpal tunnel?

- Flexor digitorium profundus (four tendons)
- Flexor digitorum superficialis (four tendons)
- Flexor pollicis longus (one tendon)
- Median nerve
- Flexor carpi radialis (split ligament)

What are the attachments of the flexor retinaculum?

- Pisiform, hook of hamate (ulnar)
- Tubercle of scaphoid, ridge of trapezium (radial)

What structures are at risk?

- Palmaris longus
- Palmar cutaneous branch of median nerve

- Recurrent motor branch of median nerve
- Superficial branch of the radial artery
- Ulnar artery and nerve
- Palmar arch (superficial and deep) (Figure 11.16)

Appendectomy

How would you perform an appendectomy?

- Ensure you are performing the correct operation for the correct reasons (re-take history, re-examine the patient and confirm the appropriate imaging).
- Obtain informed consent and mark the correct side (right-side).
- WHO checklist.
- Supine position.
- General anaesthesia, supine position.
- Standard preparation and drape (whole abdomen).
- IV antibiotics (cefuroxime and metronidazole).
- Access to peritoneal cavity.
- Lanz incision (runs along Langer's lines, 1–2 cm medial to anterior superior iliac spine [ASIS]) over McBurney's point.
- Dissect through the subcutaneous fat and fascia, down to external oblique aponeurosis.
- Make incision through the aponeurosis, parallel to the wound incision.
- Split muscle fibres of external oblique, internal oblique and transversus abdominis.
- Open peritoneum.

Steps:

- Swab (MC&S).
- Inspect caecum and small bowel for other pathology.

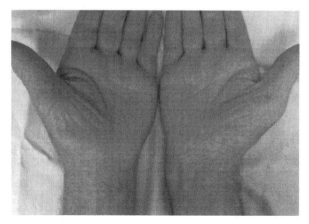

Figure 11.16 Thenar muscle wasting in carpal tunnel syndrome.

- Meckel's diverticulum, caecal tumour, ovarian masses (ovarian cysts or tumours) and the fallopian tube (ectopic pregnancy).
- Identify the taeniae coli on caecum and follow down to appendix.
- Clip and divide vessels on the mesoappendix (Figure 11.18).
- Apply Dunhill forceps to base.
- Surgical tie to the base and then divide base.
- Purse string is applied to the caecum and bury the stump.
- Perform a peritoneal lavage with betadine to reduce risk of infection.
- With a new set instruments, close the wound in layers with an absorbable suture (e.g. vicryl).

What is the difference between the Gridiron/McBurney's and Lanz incisions?

Gridiron/McBurney's incision

- Surface marking one-third of way along an imaginary line joining the right ASIS and the umbilicus. An incision is made perpendicular to this line.

Lanz incision

- This incision is used more commonly as it results in better cosmetic results. This incision is made horizontally over McBurney's point (Figures 11.17).

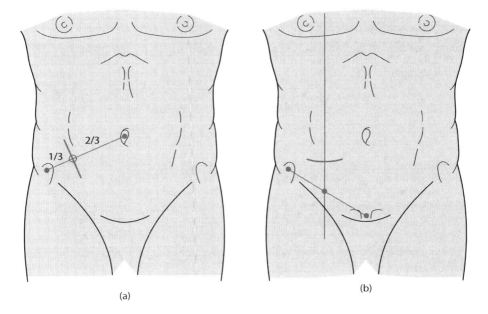

Figure 11.17 (a) Gridiron incision for appendicitis, at right angles to a line joining the anterior superior iliac spine and umbilicus, centred on McBurney's point. (b) Transverse or skin crease (Lanz) incision for appendicitis, 2 cm below the umbilicus, centred on the mid–clavicular–mid-inguinal line. (Courtesy of Professor M Earley, FRSCI, Dublin, Ireland.)

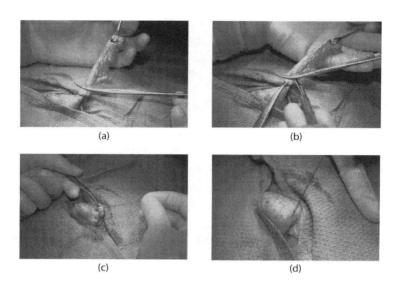

(a) (b)

(c) (d)

Figure 11.18 (a) Mesoappendix divided between artery forceps and ligated. (b) Appendix crushed and ligated at its base and about to be divided. (c) 'Z' suture inserted prior to inversion of the appendiceal stump. (d) Appendiceal stump inverted, the 'Z' suture having been tied.

Fasciotomy

What are the compartments of the lower limb?

Compartment	Muscles	Neurovascular structures
Anterior compartment	Tibialis anterior, extensor hallucis longus, extensor digitorum longus and peroneus tertius	Deep peroneal nerve and anterior tibial vessels
Lateral compartment	Fibularis longus and brevis	Superficial peroneal nerve and fibular artery
Deep posterior compartment	Tibialis posterior, flexor hallucis longus, flexor digitorum longus and popliteus	Tibial nerve, posterior tibial artery and posterior tibial vessels such as the fibular artery
Superficial posterior compartment	Gastrocnemius, soleus and plantaris	Tibial nerve, medial sural cutaneous nerve, posterior tibial artery

When do you suspect compartment syndrome?

- Pain out of proportion to injury and unresponsive to analgesia
- Pain on passive stretching of the individual compartment
- Paralysis, paraesthesia and pulselessness are late signs

How do you treat compartment syndrome?

This is a surgical emergency.

- All circumferential dressings, including plasters, should be removed at once.
- Perform an urgent fasciotomy of all compartments.
- Double incision technique with perifibular fasciotomy.
- Decompress superficial and deep posterior compartments through a medial longitudinal incision placed 1–2 cm posterior to the medial border of tibia (keep anterior to posterior tibial artery to avoid injury to perforating vessels that supply local flaps).
- Decompress anterior and lateral compartments through a longitudinal incision 2 cm lateral to anterior tibial border (Figures 11.19 and 11.20).

Hernia repair

What types are the different types of inguinal hernias?

- Indirect
- Direct
- Combined (Pantaloon)

How do you differentiate between direct and indirect inguinal hernias?

Clinically

- Finger over midpoint of inguinal canal (deep ring)
- If swelling is controlled then it is an indirect hernia
- If hernia bulges medial to finger (through the muscle wall of inguinal canal) then it is a direct hernia

At surgery

- Relationship to inferior epigastric artery
- Direct hernia sac lies medial to the artery
- Indirect hernia sac lies lateral to the artery

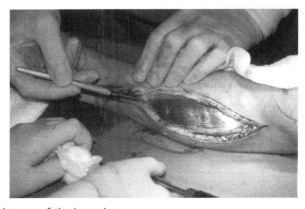

Figure 11.19 Fasciotomy of the lower leg.

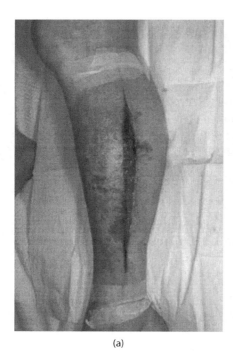

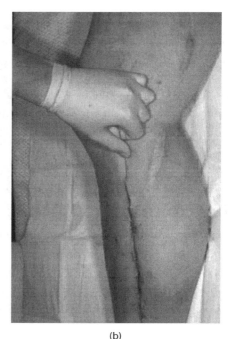

(a)   (b)

Figure 11.20 Delayed primary closure of fasciotomy wound.

Mnemonic is MD – *Medial* to artery is a *direct* hernia.

How do you repair an indirect hernia?

- Ensure you are performing the correct operation for the correct reasons (re-take history, re-examine the patient and confirm the appropriate imaging).
- Obtain informed consent and mark the correct side.
- WHO checklist.
- General anaesthesia and supine position.
- Standard preparation and drape.
- Antibiotics at induction.
- Incision (transverse skin incision in groin crease overlying the hernia, through the subcutaneous fat, Scarpa's fascia to external oblique aponeurosis).
- Expose superficial ring and open inguinal canal to expose spermatic cord and its contents.
- Examine the spermatic cord to identify hernia sac.
- Dissect hernial sac off spermatic cord.
- Cremasteric vessels may need to be ligated and divided to gain access and achieve haemostasis.
- Open sac to identify bowel or omentum.
- Transfix and excise the sac.

- Repair and reinforce weakened posterior wall of inguinal canal with a prolene mesh by the Lichtenstein technique.
- Closure in layers (vicryl) (Figure 11.21).

What are the boundaries of the inguinal canal?

Boundaries of inguinal canal

	Superior wall (roof): Internal oblique Transversus abdominis	

Anterior wall:
Aponeurosis of external oblique
Aponeurosis of internal oblique
  (lateral third of canal only)
Superficial inguinal ring (medial
  third of canal only)
	(Inguinal canal)	Posterior wall:
		Transversalis fascia
		Conjoint tendon (medial
		  third of canal only)
		Deep inguinal ring
		  (lateral third of canal
		  only)

	Inferior wall (floor):
	Inguinal ligament
	Lacunar ligament (medial
	  third of canal only)
	Iliopubic tract (lateral
	  third of canal only)	

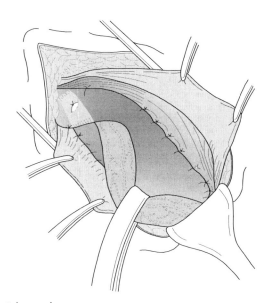

Figure 11.21 Lichtenstein repair.

Thyroidectomy

- Ensure you are performing the correct operation for the correct reasons (re-take history, re-examine the patient and confirm the appropriate imaging).
- Obtain informed consent and mark the correct side.
- WHO checklist.
- General anaesthesia, supine position with shoulder roll and head ring.
- Collar incision two fingers' breadth above sternal notch.
- Elevate flap in subplatysma plane to level of superior border of thyroid cartilage, which is superficial to anterior jugular vein.
- Dissect in the midline to retract the strap muscles.
- Ligate middle thyroid vein.
- Dissect superior pole, ligate and divide the superior pedicle. Double tie and transfix the superior pole.
- Mobilise inferior pole.
- Identify the recurrent laryngeal nerve – Use inferior thyroid artery as a landmark.
- Ligate the inferior thyroid artery – Ideally medially in order to preserve the parathyroid gland blood supply.
- Follow the recurrent laryngeal nerve until it enters under cricopharyngeus.
- Remove gland.
- Obtain haemostasis and insert a drain.
- Close strap muscles over trachea (to prevent tracheal tethering to the skin).
- Close wound.

What is the arterial supply and venous drainage to the thyroid gland?

Arterial supply:

- Superior thyroid artery (external carotid artery)
- Inferior thyroid artery (subclavian artery-thyrocervical trunk)
- Midline thyroid ima artery (aortic arch in ~10% of people)

Venous drainage:

- Superior thyroid vein (facial or internal jugular vein)
- Middle thyroid vein (internal jugular vein)
- Inferior thyroid vein (brachiocephalic vein)

What are the post-operative complications of a thyroidectomy?

- Scar
- Haemorrhage
- Infection
- Respiratory obstruction
- Recurrent laryngeal nerve paralysis and voice change
- Thyroid insufficiency
- Parathyroid insufficiency
- Thyrotoxic crisis (storm) (Figure 11.22)

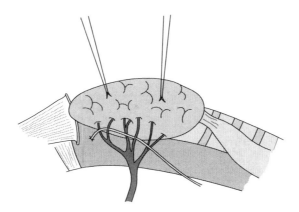

Figure 11.22 Identification of the recurrent laryngeal nerve. Note how rotating the gland medially anteriorly kinks the nerve that is normally intimately related to the terminal branches of the inferior thyroid artery.

CHAPTER 12:
COMMUNICATION SKILLS
FOR THE MRCS OSCE

The communication skills OSCE

Communication skills framework model

Top tips

THE COMMUNICATION SKILLS OSCE

Doctors must communicate effectively with patients, relatives, colleagues and other professionals from an entire spectrum of socio-economic and cultural backgrounds. This requires skill in verbal, non-verbal, written and telephone etiquette to quickly establish an appropriate and productive rapport to convey and receive information in a structured and comprehensive manner. Assessment of communication skills is a major feature of the Membership of the Royal College of Surgeons (MRCS) objective structured clinical examination (OSCE) and should not be underestimated. Good communication skills are often second nature to caring, dynamic and articulate doctors, however, as with any exam there are effective techniques to maximise success in such cases and vignettes.

Communication skills OSCE stations are identical in length to the other stations (9 minutes) and may be manned or unmanned. The unmanned stations are usually written tasks such as writing a referral letter using a patient's medical notes. The manned stations generally begin with an opening minute for preparation of the clinical scenario with the information provided, followed by 9 minutes to act out the task. This could include discussion with a patient, relative or another health-care professional.

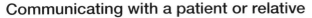

Communicating with a patient or relative

Typical scenarios include taking a focussed history, breaking bad news, explaining a procedure or obtaining consent and dealing with angry or upset patients and relatives (complaints).

Communicating with another health professional

Typical scenarios include writing a referral letter or discharge summary using clinical case notes and making a direct referral face to face or over the phone.

It is clear that in order to complete these tasks effectively, adequate medical knowledge is essential. However, it is important to remember that it is the communication skills aspect that is being primarily assessed. With this in mind, there are some useful framework models that can be applied to these stations, which always begins with meticulous systematic preparation.

COMMUNICATION SKILLS FRAMEWORK MODEL

The communication skills OSCE is very much run by you and you should therefore have a structured, logical framework or game plan specific to this part of the exam. Here is a suggested format.

1. Preparation

   - This involves the preparation time to work through the vignette registering the task at hand and the salient information required from the material provided.
   - You should map out the scenario including opening statements to the examiner such as 'leaving your pager with a colleague to avoid being disturbed', 'selecting a private, tranquil room for the consultation' etc.
   - You should re-arrange the chairs to ensure that you are positioned in a non-defensive and approachable manner rather than across a desk. This demonstrates to the examiners that you have insight into social dynamics before you even begin the consultation.

2. Introduction

   - First impressions are critical and can set the mood and fate for the remainder of the OSCE station.
   - The patient, relative or colleague should be greeted by providing your name and position and also by inviting them to introduce themselves by name and affiliation to the patient (or position in the case of another health-care professional).

- It is mandatory to state that you would ensure you have consent from the patient concerned if you are communicating with extended family members.
- The patient or relative should be asked if they wish to be alone or accompanied by a friend, family member or nurse before proceeding any further.

3. **Consultation**

- This should commence with setting the scene and establishing what the patient, friend or other health-care professional understands about the current medical condition.
- Use of appropriate verbal and non-verbal communication techniques is vital to avoid misunderstandings through miscommunication.
- Language should be pitched appropriately to the person in question and so medical jargon may be justified when communicating with a colleague but is deemed inappropriate when communicating with a patient or relative.
- The sequence of open-ended questions, followed by direct questions and then closed questions usually works well in most situations. This engages the person early on by empowering them in the conversation, building trust and a good rapport.
- Open questioning should address the person's ideas, concerns and expectations 'ICE'. The nature of these obviously varies according to the person. For example, a patient may be hiding a plethora of psychosocial issues whereas a busy intensivist might be trying to deal with the pressures of multiple teams fighting for that last intensive care unit (ICU) bed.
- Revealing the person's underlying agenda is often the key in the art of persuasion, as this then allows you to understand where they are coming from and thus develops convincing arguments. For example, you might be consenting a patient for an operation whose close family member died on the operating table. Alternatively, you might be referring to the intensivist who will be waiting to hear clinical evidence that meets ICU admission criteria before accepting the referral.
- Body language and simple courtesy and etiquette are important aids to allow free-flow of communication. Defensive positions, e.g. arms crossed and lack of eye contact are often inhibitory to the consultation, whereas demonstrating active interest by repeating the salient points of what has been communicated and seeking clarification, tend to facilitate the process.
- Illustrations (e.g. pictures and diagrams) and patient information leaflets are helpful aids to demonstrate the important features of your discussion, which the patient or relative may take away with them. Other powerful tools include the use of silences and pauses to give the person space to think and express their true concerns.
- The power of smiling (if appropriate) cannot be underestimated as it removes intimidation and fear and introduces an air of calm and welcome. If, however,

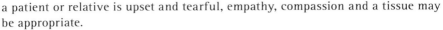

a patient or relative is upset and tearful, empathy, compassion and a tissue may be appropriate.

- Use words which the patient will understand (e.g. 'cancer') and avoid medial jargon (e.g. 'mitotic lesion', 'malignancy', 'growth') when breaking the bad news. Bear in mind that patients are often in a state of shock on hearing such loaded words and may not absorb any further information from that point onwards.
- Gauging a patient's non-verbal communication is often more pertinent than their verbal communication and in some cases it may be appropriate to continue the consultation another time.
- If a person is angry or aggressive, it is best to remain calm and ask them to explain their reasons so that you may understand their concerns. You should then re-iterate what you have understood back to them and then offer a plan in an attempt to ameliorate the situation. Of course, if there has been a misunderstanding or mistake, you should apologise.
- It is important to stress that clinical knowledge is required to provide the medium through which communication skills is being assessed. However, in areas beyond your expertise it is correct and right to admit incomplete knowledge and state that you will consult a senior colleague or seek advice from experts in other disciplines, i.e. the multidisciplinary approach.

4. Consolidation

- You should ask the other person to repeat back what he or she has understood so far, which may then highlight whether there is any confusion or any further issues to address.
- If there is confusion, miscommunication or disagreement, these must be addressed at this time using 'ICE' once again and then focussing in on the problem. This is obligatory when obtaining consent from a patient for a procedure.
- A patient has the right to refuse treatment if he or she has proven to understand the facts.
- There may be times where an immediate solution or compromise cannot be reached and scheduling a second meeting to discuss the matter further may well be the best option.

5. Conclusion

- You should summarise what has been communicated and provide an agreed management plan.
- Your name, position and contact details should be given to the patient, relative or colleague for the future and a follow-up appointment or meeting can be arranged.
- Finally, you should thank the person for their time and close the session appropriately, e.g. 'been a pleasure speaking with you', 'I hope that helps, we can discuss it further next time' etc.

TOP TIPS

Taking a history

This should include the eight classic features:

1. Personal details – Name, age, sex and occupation

2. PC (presenting complaint)

3. HoPc (history of presenting complaint) – Onset, duration, character, associated features, risk factors, system-specific history, investigations and treatment to date

4. PMHx (past medical history), PSHx (past surgical history)

5. DHx (drug history) and allergies

6. FHx (family history)

7. SOHx (social and occupational history) – Including alcohol (e.g. pancreatitis), smoking (smoking-related cancers), foreign travel (e.g. diarrhoea), asbestos exposure (e.g. mesothelioma)

8. SR (systems review) – Cardiovascular, respiratory, gastrointestinal, urological, neurological and musculoskeletal

- A useful mnemonic for breaking bad news is '**SPIKES**' (Buckman et al.):
  S   Set stage and setting – Confidential.
  P   Patient perception – 'ICE'.
  I   Invitation – Are they prepared to discuss?
  K   Knowledge – Their understanding.
  E   Explore emotions and empathise – Create space for reaction and listen.
  S   Strategy and summary – Discuss management plan and give contact details.

- A useful mnemonic when consenting a patient for a procedure is '**CONSENTS**'.
  C   Condition and natural history – Explain the clinical condition and prognosis.
  O   Options and alternatives – No treatment, conservative, medical, radiological, surgical.
  N   Name of procedure – Official title and practically what it entails.
  S   Side effects/complications – Anaesthetic, infection, bleeding, recurrence, others, e.g. stoma formation etc.
  E   Extra procedures – E.g. drain, nasogastric (NG) tube, catheter, patient-controlled analgesia (PCA) insertion; stoma formation; blood transfusion etc.
  N   Named person operating – Plus assistants.
  T   Trial and training – If part of a research trial or presence of any students.
  S   Second opinion – A second opinion may be obtained prior to consenting.

Abbreviations

5-HT	5-hydroxytryptamine
AAA	Abdominal aortic aneurysm
AAFB	Acid–alcohol-fast bacilli
ABG	Arterial blood gas
ABPI	Ankle-brachial pressure index
ACE	Angiotensin-converting enzyme
ACJ	Acromioclavicular joint
ACTH	Adrenocorticotropic hormone
ADH	Anti-diuretic hormone
AF	Atrial fibrillation
ALP	Alkaline phosphatase
ALT	Alanine aminotransferase
ARDS	Acute respiratory distress syndrome
AS	Ankylosing spondylitis
ASA	American Society of Anesthesiologists
ASIS	Anterior superior iliac spine
AST	Aspartate aminotransferase
ATLS	Advanced trauma life support
AXR	Abdominal x-ray
BCC	Basal cell carcinoma
BE	Base excess
BIPAP	Bi-level positive airway pressure
BM	Blood glucose
BMI	Body mass index
BP	Blood pressure
CABG	Coronary artery bypass graft
CBD	Common bile duct
CCF	Congestive cardiac failure
CD	Crohn's disease
CEA	Carcinoembryonic antigen
CMV	Cytomegalovirus
CNS	Central nervous system
CO	Cardiac output
COPD	Chronic obstructive pulmonary disease
CPAP	Continuous positive airway pressure
CPE	Carbapenem-resistant Enterobacteriaceae
CRP	C-reactive protein
CSF	Cerebrospinal fluid
CT	Computed tomography
CTPA	Computed tomography pulmonary angiogram
CVA	Cerebrovascular accident
CVP	Central venous pressure

CXR	Chest x-ray
DIC	Disseminated intravascular coagulation
DIPJ	Distal interphalangeal joint
DRE	Digital rectal examination
DVT	Deep vein thrombosis
EBV	Epstein–Barr virus
ECF	Extracellular fluid
ECG	Electrocardiogram
ECHO	Echocardiogram
EHL	Extensor hallucis longus
EPL	Extensor pollicis longus
ERCP	Endoscopic retrograde cholangio-pancreatography
ESR	Erythrocyte sedimentation rate
FBC	Full blood count
FCU	Flexor carpi ulnaris
FDP	Flexor digitorum profundus
FDS	Digitorum superficialis
FEV	Forced expiratory volume
FFD	Fixed flexion deformity
FFP	Fresh frozen plasma
FNAC	Fine needle aspiration cytology
FPL	Flexor pollicis longus
FRED	Facial nerve, retromandibular vein, external carotid artery and deep
FSH	Follicle stimulating hormone
FVC	Forced vital capacity
G&S	Group and save
GA	General anaesthetic
GCS	Glasgow Coma Scale
GH	Growth hormone
GI	Gastrointestinal
GMC	General Medical Council
GP	General practitioner
GTN	Glyceryl trinitrate
Hb	Haemoglobin
HBV	Hepatitis B virus
HCC	Hepatocellular carcinoma
HCG	Human chorionic gonadotrophin
HCV	Hepatitis C virus
HHV	Human herpes virus
HIV	Human immunodeficiency virus
HPV	Human papillomavirus
HR	Heart rate
HRT	Hormone replacement therapy
HSV	Herpes simplex virus
HTLV	Human T-cell leukaemia virus

IBD	Inflammatory bowel disease
ICD	Implantable cardiac defibrillator
ICP	Intracranial pressure
ICU	Intensive care unit
IHD	Ischaemic heart disease
IM	Intramuscular
IPJ	Interphalangeal joint
ITP	Idiopathic thrombocytopaenic purpura
ITU	Intensive treatment unit
IV	Intravenous
IVDU	Intravenous drug user
IVI	Intravenous infusion
JACCOL	Jaundice, anaemia, cyanosis, clubbing, oedema, lymphadenopathy
JPS	Joint position sense
JVP	Jugular venous pressure
LDH	Lactate dehydrogenase
LFT	Liver function test
LH	Luteinizing hormone
LHS	Left hand side
LIF	Left iliac fossa
LMN	Lower motor neuron
LMW	Low molecular weight
LUQ	Left upper quadrant
MCP	Metacarpophalangeal joint
MDT	Multi-disciplinary team
MEN	Multiple endocrine neoplasia
MI	Myocardial infarction
MR	Magnetic resonance
MRC	Medical Research Council
MRCS	Membership of the Royal College of Surgeons
MRI	Magnetic resonance imaging
MRSA	Methicillin resistant *Staphylococcus aureus*
NBM	Nil by mouth
NG	Nasogastric
NHS	National Health Service
NICE	National Institute for Clinical Excellence
NO	Nitric oxide
NPC	Nasopharyngeal carcinoma
NSAID	Non-steroidal anti-inflammatory drug
OA	Osteoarthritis
OCP	Oral contraceptive pill
OGD	Oesophago-gastro-duodenoscopy
OSCE	Objective structured clinical examination
PBC	Primary biliary cirrhosis
PCA	Patient controlled analgesia

PE	Pulmonary embolus
PEEP	Positive end expiratory pressure
PEFR	Peak expiratory flow rate
PEG	Percutaneous endoscopic gastrostomy
PEP	Post-exposure prophylaxis
PIPJ	Proximal interphalangeal joint
PNS	Peripheral nervous system
PR	Per rectum
PSA	Prostate-specific antigen
PUO	Pyrexia of unknown origin
PVD	Peripheral vascular disease
RIF	Right iliac fossa
RR	Respiratory rate
RUQ	Right upper quadrant
SCC	Squamous cell carcinoma
SCJ	Sternoclavicular joint
SFJ	Sapheno-femoral junction
SIJ	Sacro-iliac joint
SIRS	Systemic inflammatory response syndrome
SLE	Systemic lupus erythematosus
SVC	Superior vena cava
TB	Tuberculosis
TED	Thromboembolic deterrent
TGF	Transforming growth factor
TIBC	Total iron binding capacity
TNF	Tumour necrosis factor
TNM	Tumour, node and metastasis
TPR	Total peripheral resistance
TRAM	Transverse rectus abdominis flap
TSH	Thyroid-stimulating hormone
U&E	Urea and electrolyte
UC	Ulcerative colitis
UMN	Upper motor neuron
USS	Ultrasound scan
UTI	Urinary tract infection
VATS	Video-assisted thoracoscopic surgery
VRE	Vancomycin resistant Enterococci
WCC	White cell count
WHO	World Health Organisation

List of figures

is rolled and a sliding board (arrow) is placed under the patient and undersheet or canvas, which will allow the patient to slide across to the bed in a controlled fashion. Care is being taken by all of the team members to protect the whole patient.

Chapter 5

Chapter 11

Index